You Don't Have To Die When Your Doctor Says

You Don't Have To Die When Your Doctor Says

A practical guide to living with grace and joy in the face of a terminal prognosis.

(...and who doesn't have a terminal prognosis?)

David Elliot

Primary
Press

Whitianga • Whenuakite

Original copyright © 2009 by David Elliot

Published and Distributed in New Zealand by

Primary Press

320 Boatharbour Rd. RD1 Whitianga. NZ

www.survivecancer.info

ISBN 978-0-473-15016-7

Cover design and photography by David Elliot
Author portrait by Stephanie Muir

Preface

This book will not cure you of cancer or a terminal disease; it does not contain any miracle cures, therapies being suppressed by the American Medical Association, cancer curing diets or secrets. What this book does contain is viewpoints that may help you create faith in your own healing ability and inspire you to engage your will and live as fully and for as long as possible. My intention is to challenge you to live with grace and joy in the face of a terminal prognosis, to be the most you can be and/or to die trying.

The information contained within this book has no scientific basis whatsoever and is not intended to be taken in any way as clinically proven or evidence based fact. The viewpoints expressed are created from my own experience of being diagnosed with a 'terminal' cancer, from supporting other sufferers and from my experience and training as an Avatar® Master.

If you have been diagnosed with cancer, or any other serious disease or disability or have been given a medical death sentence then you are off the map, beyond the safe shores of science; here there be monsters! But this is also the doorway to belief, faith and personal responsibility.

This Book is dedicated to all those who helped me when I could not help myself.

Whitianga and Hahei ambulance staff.
Thames emergency department and ward staff.
Hamilton neurosurgery and oncology staff.
My family and friends.

Thank You.

Last Update. 30/January/2010

This is my last update because I realise that I am now dying of brain cancer. It has been 25 months since I was initially diagnosed with gmb and considering that my prognosis was that I had a 90% chance of being dead within two years, I've done all right.

Just over a week ago I had a MRI which showed that the tumour has grown through a large area of the left side of my brain. I am experiencing constant headaches, tiredness, difficulty reading and talking, memory loss and physical limitations.

To recap, I have had brain surgery twice (on the initial tumour and a recurrence) chemotherapy and radiotherapy. Now I have a third occurrence which has been growing in my left parietal area since august 2001. I decided not to have a third surgical intervention so really had no medical actions at all.

Through out my experience of having cancer I have maintained (most times) a positive attitude and put my attention towards the possibility that I will survive as well as also accounting for possibility the cancer will be fatal. Now that, baring an absolute miracle, I realise that my death is only a matter of time, maybe I will have a few weeks or health or maybe not.

If you are facing a 'fatal' disease, I feel for you from my heart. All I can say for you is be strong, feel all your experiences and love. Through the past two years I have had to learn so much, but it has been OK, even the fear and loss and suffering.

Even though my life is being daily reduced, my capacity to love is only growing. Yes I am soon leaving my family, my loving wife and my children (fortunately young independent and amazing girls) which is my greatest source of sadness, but I am so blessed by what I have had and still have, that this sadness is just part of bitterness and sweetness that we need in life.

My book is not an authority on how to survive brain cancer, but I hope that it can be of some help to any other person who finds themselves facing the fear of a terminal prognosis. It is very scary but I believe that death is not so terrible. We will all face this portal but let us not let it cause such fear that we forget to enjoy even a moment of life.

Thank you and may your days be full of joy.

David Elliot.

Contents

Pain, what it means and how we deal with it.

Being diagnosed

90% chance of being dead in 2 years!

Searching for answers

Getting an upgrade and choosing chemo

Updates

Introduction

You Don't Have To Die When Your Doctor Says is a book about the power of belief in the context of a serious disease or medical death sentence. In many ways I have written this book for myself, but if you are experiencing a diagnosis of cancer or have been told you only have so long to live then I have also written it for you (and that's why it's a fairly brief book!)

I have been living with a medical death sentence since January 2008 when I was diagnosed with glioma multiforme blastoma stage 4 and told I had only a 10% chance of living two years. Writing this book has helped me clarify my beliefs; my belief in myself and in my understanding of the role of belief in healing and the beliefs that underpin both allopathic and alternative treatments. Often I have had to take my own advice. There have been times when I have been feeling sorry for myself or using my situation as an excuse and I have had to remember what I have written and live up to my words.

I have come to realise my diagnosis is not a tragedy and my possible death is also not something to worry about. I have also come to believe I don't need to conform to mortality statistics. You might find it hard to believe, but most days I don't worry about having cancer or dying at all.

Throughout the course of this disease I have had to face my mortality and reassess my values. I now know I am loved and supported by my family, my friends, my Avatar sanga, my community and my universe (which includes an undefined sense of God). Grappling with the issues of my death has brought me to a greater appreciation of my life. Before my illness I was still uncommitted, a stranger to faith and still seeking. Now I am found; I have found myself and I have found peace and joy.

If my words can help you through your turbulent times and move you a single step closer to peace and joy then I am satisfied.

Please use this book to explore your beliefs. Throughout the text there are questions for you to consider; please take the time to actually answer them. Even better; get a notebook and write your answers down. It is from your interaction with the text that you will gain the most insight into your own beliefs about your healing. If you only read the text, you might gain some insight into my beliefs but that will not be as helpful as answering the questions and gaining insight into your beliefs. Your beliefs, not mine, are creating your experience. It's changing your beliefs that will change your experience.

It is not my intention to deter you from any course of medical treatment; I support any choice you make. It is my intention to hold you in the highest regard and acknowledge you as an amazing creative being. You are a manifestation of God, of the creative force of the universe and you have it within you to heal.

Some may say I am being a bit previous, considering myself a survivor when I haven't yet lived past my predicted use-by date but my viewpoint is that success isn't a result or a destination; it's a way of being. I am deciding right now that I am a survivor. Waiting to see if I survive and then celebrating success implies a lack of belief. Every day I draw breath, I am a survivor! Every day I can celebrate the success of being alive. It's a great way to live.

Chapter 1

The Diagnosis

The mistakes made by doctors are innumerable. They err habitually on the side of optimism as to treatment, of pessimism as to the outcome.
Marcel Proust

Any medical story starts with the diagnosis. Granted, there is always something going on prior to that occurrence; some symptoms or emergency which takes you to the doctor or the hospital in the first place, but until the diagnosis is made, all is conjecture, worry and confusion. Then comes the time when you are sitting in your hospital bed in pain and worry, with your loved ones in attendance, and the doctor utters those fateful words: 'I am sorry....*insert your name* ... but you have...*insert your fearful malady...*'

This diagnosis is the start of your new life and, inevitably, the first thing you want to know is how long your new life is going to be? So you ask the doctor.

This is a mistake!

Thinking that your doctor is God and can predict your future is a reasonable mistake to make. Doctors can appear Godlike in their apparent abilities to give and take life. They routinely perform miracles and bestow blessings, but still, doctors are as mortal and human as the rest of us. They also make mistakes.

No matter what you are suffering from, no doctor can tell you how long you have to live. They can tell you what they would expect based on their previous experience and they can back up their estimates with clinical data from previous cases but this information is not really about you, it's about their beliefs about the disease and it's about other people's experiences.

To ask the question is to give your authority away and the answer, no matter how compassionately given or factually based is a figurative nail in your coffin.

You might be told you have a few years or it might be a few weeks but whatever the numbers, a medical prediction is the scientific equivalent of the witchdoctor's curse. The bone has been pointed and if you are to survive, sooner or later, you are going to have to lift this curse.

If you did ask, take it back. If you were told without asking, you don't need to believe the answer; it's just the opinion of someone in a white coat.

Exercising your right to choose is an act of human dignity. I'm with the Bible on this one; we have the freedom of choice. Does that mean we choose and then wait to see if God decides to grant us, or not grant us, what we chose? I don't think so. What sort of choice is that? I believe God (or the universe, however you like to think of it) empowers and supports all our choices. The problem is that we make a lot of our choices automatically and unconsciously, based on old beliefs and assumptions we have forgotten and that are no longer serving us

So now, in the present moment, choose again.

Decide for yourself how long you are going to live. The worst that can happen is that you will be wrong and die before your time, big deal, at least you acted with spirit.

No matter how you were told, receiving the news, even if you already suspected it, is always a shock. We are all going to die. You know this. So why is it such a shock when you get reminded of the inevitable?

You sit there stunned and reeling, numbed by the news that your body is mortal. Then the thinking kicks in and you begin worrying about the future. Questions parade past your awareness: When will I die? How much will I suffer? Will I be a burden on my loved ones? How did this happen to me?

It's as if you never thought you would ever die at all. All your plans and actions have been based on the belief of your continued existence. You know other people suffer and die but that's not really the same is it? Other people have terminal diseases, but not you! It just doesn't feel right. Surely it's some kind of mistake!

There can be many different reactions to the initial terminal prognosis; we can take the news with resigned acceptance and dignity or with defiant refusal. Denial is to be expected and even relief is not out of the question. Anger, sadness and grief are all possible responses. Quite likely you will experience every possible response as time goes by, repeatedly. There is no right or wrong response to the news; there is just what you feel, but at some point you are going to have to accept your situation and begin to consider what you are going to do about it.

Examining your beliefs, about the prognosis, about the disease and about your ability to heal, would be a good place to start.

Chapter 2

Are Beliefs Important for Healing?

*The beliefs you truly hold, the ones you've decided to believe, your faith, will
cause you to create or attract the experiences which will verify them.*
Harry Palmer

Many people, including many doctors, will tell you that what
you believe will not have any effect on the course of your
illness or your likelihood of experiencing a cure. But that's
what they believe. What do you believe? What do you want to
believe?

Let's explore this a little more; what if they are right? Well,
you can at least entertain the idea that your beliefs and
attitudes will have an effect on your perceptions and
experiences even if not your life expectancy. Consider how you
felt when you were told that you had cancer or a terminal
disease. What caused your response of worry and fear? All
that happened was that someone you trusted gave you some
information and you believed it to be true. Nothing changed
about your condition or your symptoms but suddenly you felt
the bottom fall out of your world. This is the power of belief.
So changing your belief will, at the very least, change how you
feel.

So given that your life expectancy is predicted to be severely reduced, how do you want to feel? For a few moments, focus you attention on the following beliefs:

- My condition is incurable.
- No one can help me.
- It doesn't matter what I do.
- It won't make a difference what I believe.
- I am sick and am going to die.

How do you feel?

Now focus your attention on these beliefs:

- I am loved and supported.
- There are things I can do to facilitate healing.
- What I believe makes a difference.
- I have a medical condition but I can heal.
- My body manifested this so my body can cure itself.

How do you feel?

Do you want to spend the rest of your days exhausted by fear and despair or inspired by hope and a strong intention to grow in health? Which attitude will be most likely to induce you to research alternative cures or find inspired health practitioners? Which attitude will make you more receptive to the effects of a good diet? Which attitude will boost your immune system? It's beginning to look as though your beliefs might just have an effect on your chances of survival and quality of life after all.

Bernie Siegel. M.D believes in the power of belief in healing. In his book *Love, Medicine and Miracles* he writes:

'To become exceptional in caring for the body, one must take stock of the beliefs one has about it, especially those so ingrained that they are normally unconscious. If a person can turn from predicting illness to anticipating recovery, the foundation of a cure is laid.'

Dr. Siegel goes on to illustrate the power of belief as exemplified by the story of Mr. Wright, a client of psychologist Bruno Klopfer in 1957.

Mr. Wright had far-advanced lymphosarcoma with tumors the size of oranges in his neck, groin, chest and armpits. He had already exhausted all known treatments and was expected to die of his disease. Mr. Wright had not given up hope though and when he heard of a new drug called Krebiozen he begged so hard to be included in the trial that he was given a shot of the new drug even though he didn't qualify as a study subject. Dr. Klopfer expected Mr. Wright to be dead the following morning but was amazed to find him out of his bed and chatting happily. With continued treatments of Krebiozen Mr. Wright's tumors melted away within a few days even though the other study subjects showed no such improvements. Mr. Wright was discharged within 10 days. Within months, however, conflicting reports began to appear in the media about the effectiveness of the drug and Mr. Wright relapsed to his original state and returned to hospital depressed and once more near death.

At this point Dr. Klopfer assured Mr. Wright that the bad press was due to the early shipments of the drug deteriorating during transit and promised to treat him with some fresh, extra potent Krebiozen. Mr. Wright's attitude became once more positive and he responded to the drug again with amazing results, except the injections he received were actually only water. This could have possibly been a happy story except that it seems that Mr. Wright was never told that his miracle cure was really created by his belief in a non existent drug. Sadly after reading further reports on the worthlessness of Krebiozen, Mr Wright was re-admitted to the hospital in extremis, his faith was gone, his last hope vanished, and he succumbed in less than two days.

Deepak Chopra, medical doctor and author, tells a similar story in *Quantum Healing*. A patient who presented with chest pain. After x-ray and biopsy it was confirmed that the patient had a large tumor between his lungs diagnosed as oat-cell carcinoma, an extremely deadly, very fast growing malignancy. The patient refused treatment and went home but returned again, 8 years later, with a similar growth in his neck. His doctor was amazed to find him alive and with no trace of lung cancer. He considered that, normally, 99.99 percent of untreated patients would have died within six months. When asked what he had done about his previous cancer the patient replied that he had done nothing, just decided he was not going to let himself die from cancer and that he may also refuse treatment with this second cancer.

As a third example of the power of belief I would like to tell you about Lolette Kuby who healed herself of breast cancer. In 1982 Lolette elected to undergo breast enhancement surgery and asked her doctor to check out a lump on her breast, 'while she was open'. The pathology lab later reported that the lump was tubular cancer of the breast and the doctor recommended immediate mastectomy. Shocked and reeling from the news, Lolette declined the appointment and went home to think about it. Over the next 6 days she spent her time in meditation and reading 'new thought' writings on Christian philosophy and self healing. On the fifth day after her diagnosis Lolette had a vision of Jesus who persuaded her to let go of her problems. She then had a vision of God a few days later. She writes:

'For weeks after the revelation, I felt as though my body was surrounded by a silvery aura and that my face shone like Moses' face when he descended from Mt. Sinai. When I looked in the mirror, I saw no aura, but I did see a countenance free from fear, one that, for the first time in my life, I truly liked. And I knew that I was healed.'

Lolette's book; *Faith and the Placebo Effect* is a compelling argument for the power of belief in self-healing.

Whether or not you believe these examples are true is up to you. Whether you believe they are relevant to your situation is also up to you. Humans are blessed with the capacity to decide what they believe to be true and this capacity determines our reality. Personally, I think it's worth considering that my beliefs about my condition make a difference and I am happy to believe that people can experience dramatic remissions through their faith or simply because they refuse to die. My diagnosis of having a terminal disease is all the incentive I need to believe that well-being and health can be created through belief (and actions taken in alignment with positive belief).

What do you believe about your illness?

Because we are complex creatures it's quite likely that you will have lots of beliefs about your illness and about healing. Some of your beliefs could well contradict others. Some may be helpful for healing and some may be impeding. So sorting your beliefs out and having a good look at them could be very revealing.

On a piece of paper or in your journal, list all the beliefs that come to you when you are feeling down, when you feel hopeless and just want to give up. Include beliefs that you know are true, i.e that you consider to be facts, and beliefs that you know aren't true but you find yourself thinking them anyway. Include beliefs you are reluctant to express to others or wouldn't want to admit even to yourself.

Example: *This condition is incurable so there is no hope for me.*

Now list the beliefs that come to you when you are feeling positive. Include things you know are true and things that you suspect are wishful thinking and perhaps a bit embarrassing.

Example: *Others have cured themselves of this condition and so can I.*

Now list the beliefs you would like to hold that would help you heal, even if you don't currently think they are true.

Example: *I can change my beliefs and actions to facilitate my cure.*

If all this talk of beliefs is annoying you and you are reacting negatively to the suggestion that you are at fault for your illness; please don't think that I am suggesting that you are totally responsible for the situation you are in.

Most situations are complex and have multiple causes. Some of those causes are things that we can do nothing about, for instance, we may be genetically predisposed to a medical condition or environmental factors may be involved, or we may have suffered an accident. However, if you just focus your attention on those causes that you can do nothing about then you experience the viewpoint of victim with the consequence that there is nothing you can do to improve your life, either qualitatively or quantitatively. If, however, you are prepared to look for causes that you can take some responsibility for, then you have room to move; you no longer have the viewpoint of victim. You can make decisions and take action to improve your existence. All it takes is a lot of self-honesty and the vulnerability to allow that you may have been an active participant in your illness: now you can be an active participant in your healing.

Many health practitioners and psychologists advise against blaming the victim or encouraging people to take responsibility for their diseases. They feel it just leads to feelings of guilt and opportunities for self-recriminations that are not therapeutically healthy. I disagree with this approach because it's a soft option that avoids the power inherent in taking ownership. To say that you are not in any way responsible for your illness but that your positive attitude can have a positive influence is trying to only have one side of the coin. To discount that your negative attitude can negatively impact upon your health, by implication, discounts the value of your positive attitude.

It is true that beating yourself up and feeling guilty are not health promoting activities but this isn't what I meant by taking responsibility. Taking responsibility is simply acknowledging that certain thoughts, attitudes and actions that you have held could have contributed to the creation of the illness. If your life pattern is to then descend into self-recrimination and guilt then this is something that also needs addressing, because that pattern in itself could be part of the problem.

A recently published study carried out by a team of psychologists at the University of Pennsylvania reported that having a positive attitude gave no clinical advantage to cancer sufferers in terms of life expectancy. This was a disappointing result for the researchers, who, like many others in the healing profession, believed that a positive attitude does promote survival.

Although initially discouraging, this finding does not surprise me; I know many cancer patients with a positive attitude and outlook but who are unwilling to inspect their beliefs or take any responsibility for their condition or their healing.

Sometimes positivity is a form of pretence and masks what one is really feeling. If a person's body is wracked with disease and yet their countenance is sunny optimism then they are either a very enlightened being or they are pretending. When there is a misalignment between the body and the consciousness the resultant discord feels false. Conversely, a person who is feeling down and disheartened by the disease of their body actually has the appearance of being more real. Real positive thinking has to rest on a foundation of honesty: one has to acknowledge and own the beliefs and attitudes that could be contributing to the disease or hindering a speedy recovery and then create new, helpful beliefs.

Taking responsibility involves journeying below our habitual, surface states, of being and boldly going into the murky depths of our unconscious beliefs and attitudes and bringing them to light.

Most of what goes on in our minds and consciousness happens below our level of awareness, i.e we are unconscious of it. When psychologists talk about the subconscious, it's tempting to believe that it is a certain location or function within our mental landscape, when really it's just a catch-all term to describe whatever goes on that we are unaware of or unconscious of. The purpose of practices such as meditation, yoga and Avatar etc is to develop the ability of awareness and thus bring into consciousness that which has previously been unconscious. Yogis can consciously regulate and change bodily functions which in untrained individuals are regulated unconsciously, such as blood pressure and temperature, as an act of will. Avatar and meditation practitioners can bring to awareness beliefs, attitudes and automatic responses that have previously been unconscious. The questions and exercises in this book are designed to bring to your awareness beliefs that could be misaligned with a healthy existence so that you can do something about them.

Taking responsibility takes courage and can feel very uncomfortable at times. Taking responsibility requires actions and admissions that are challenging, but it leads to personal power. The bigger sphere of responsibility you can honestly own and accept; the more influence you will have. Whatever you deny responsibility for remains beyond your ability to change or influence.

If you still feel that you want to deny all responsibility for your illness, I empathise with you. I do know it's hard. However I won't agree with you. There are plenty of people who will quickly agree that you are not responsible for, and are helpless in the face of your disease, but they are not doing you any favours. I would rather confirm that you are an amazingly powerful creative being able to overcome any obstacle and that you, or some aspect of your higher-self, created this experience and therefore you have the power to stop creating it.

From my own experience, I know that realising, feeling and owning negative beliefs and intentions can be difficult and challenging. When I was first diagnosed I was fortunate to receive lots of loving coaching from my Avatar friends when all I wanted to do was feel sorry for myself and descend into the viewpoint of victim. They helped me to have the courage to examine my own mental blueprint of consciousness. Nearly every day for the first month of my illness they helped me unravel the turmoil of my feelings and reactions and gain a broader viewpoint on what I was experiencing. Using a very simple exercise called 'releasing fixed attention' (from ReSurfacing by Harry palmer) I explored through all the resisted layers of feelings: grief, anger, sadness, self pity etc and gained a state of emotional stability and acceptance for my condition. When I became aware of negative belief patterns, they were usually accompanied by unpleasant feelings that I had been resisting for some time, and yes there was also some self-recrimination and tears also.

But once I felt through the feelings, they passed and the negative beliefs integrated, releasing their creative energies (my attention that was invested in believing the negative

13

belief and also the attention that was invested in resisting the belief). Now my intention to live feels more real and is backed up with more of my will, rather than being self-sabotaged by denied doubts, anxious fears and the seductive thought that death could be a better option; a blessed relief from the struggles and disappointments of life. So even if I do die from this cancer, I have benefited from it already through the lessons it has brought me and the rest of my life will be lived with more love and less fear.

Changing beliefs can be as simple as making a decision. If you have a strong will or have spent time in meditation or other spiritual practices, so that you are not overly identified with your mind, then you may find it easy to simply choose to place your faith in a new belief. If, however, you are a confirmed thinker (like I was once) then you will probably find your mind demanding evidence or proof. In this case, consider your evidence for holding negative beliefs. Can you create some doubt about the veracity of the evidence? Can you find some evidence to support a new, more positive, belief? Do whatever it takes to change your mind.

As we go through this book I will show you ways to change your beliefs and present further evidence that will help you let go of the scientific paradigm that is no longer supporting you.

For a more comprehensive workout on beliefs; how they can influence your experience and how you can change your level of certainty in them, you can download the Belief Management mini course from the Avatar website, www.avatarepc.com or, better yet, get in touch with an Avatar master and schedule a free intro session.

Chapter 3

Placebo and Nocebo

The placebo effect is all in the mind.
Lolette Kuby

A placebo is defined as an inert substance given to a patient, usually during drug trials, to compare its effects with those of a 'real' drug and sometimes for the psychological benefit gained by the patient through believing that he or she is receiving real treatment. The placebo effect is a term that describes the positive therapeutic effect that the placebo can engender in the patient. It's an effect without a physical cause.

Placebos have been part of the healers' medical kit ever since there were healers and many modern medical thinkers posit that the placebo was actually the only tool that produced any health benefits prior to the advent of medical science.

In recent times when doctors became more aligned with scientific practice yet still adopted a paternalistic view towards their patients, placebos, in the form of sugar pills, were regularly dispensed as cures and were known to be particularly effective for pain relief.

In the modern era of informed consent and malpractice suits, doctors are not so keen to deliberately misinform and deceive their patients, even for good therapeutic effect, and therefore the placebo is not so deliberately used as a therapy. However, there is no reason to assume that the placebo effect is not still an integral part of every healing interaction between every therapist and their patients, no matter what modality of healing they are employing.

Drugs are prescribed and taken with the expectation, of both the doctor and the patient, that they will produce a therapeutic effect, and if an effect is achieved, it is assumed by everyone involved that the drug was the causative agent when it could of just as easily have been the expectation itself (or a combination of the two). You can exchange the word 'drug' in the above statement for any mode of alternative treatment and it will be equally as valid e.g. homeopathic tincture, color therapy session or magic potion etc. The positive expectation (ie belief) component of any cure is an immeasurable variable which can't be quantified and studied by science and is often overlooked.

Many medical writers do acknowledge the placebo effect, and quantify it as being around 30% effective in producing cures and pain relief, others claim an effectiveness of up to 80%. Trials of new pharmaceutical drugs are tested against placebos to ensure that they have a therapeutic benefit above the power of belief and suggestion alone. Though the power of belief and suggestion, labelled as 'the placebo effect' is seldom studied in its own right. Cynics point out that drug companies, who make their profits through the development of drugs that they can protect with patents, have little incentive to study something that is freely available to all.

A recent study of the placebo effect that was awarded the 2008 Ig Nobel Prize for Medicine carried out by the Massachusetts Institute of Technology demonstrated that expensive fake medicine is more effective than inexpensive fake medicine. Participants in the study were given placebo pills (inactive sugar pills) and informed that they were trialling codeine based analgesics. Half of the participants were informed that the drug had a regular price of $2.50 per pill and half that the price had been discounted to $0.10 per pill. Results showed that in the regular-price group, 85.4% of the participants experienced a mean pain reduction after taking the pill, verses 61.0% in the low-price group. What could have been different between each group? Only the value they ascribed to the medicine and therefore a mental expectation of it's effectiveness. These beliefs had a direct impact on their experience of relief from pain.

Placebo surgery has also been proven to be effective for individuals suffering from osteoarthritis of the knee. Researchers at the Houston VA Medical Centre and at Baylor College of Medicine came to this conclusion after comparing various knee treatments to placebo surgery on 180 patients with knee pain.

The patients were randomly divided into three groups. One group underwent debridement, in which the damaged or loose cartilage in the knee is surgically removed by an arthroscope; a pencil-thin tube that allows doctors to see inside the knee. The second group received arthoscopic lavage, which flushes out the bad cartilage from the healthier tissue. A third group underwent a placebo surgery. They were sedated by medication while surgeons simulated arthroscopic surgery on their knees by making small incisions on the leg, but not removing any tissue.

During a two-year follow-up, researchers found no differences among the three groups. All patients reported improvement in their symptoms of pain and ability to use their knees. Throughout the two years, patients were unaware whether they had received the 'real' or placebo surgery.

However, patients who received actual surgical treatments did not report less pain or better functioning of their knees compared to the placebo group. In fact, periodically during the follow-up, the placebo group reported a better outcome compared to the patients who underwent debridement.

The medical team who performed both the real and placebo surgeries in the study were initially very surprised with the results as they had not imagined that anything done in surgery would be beneficial from a placebo effect.

When asked why patients responded so strongly to the placebo surgery, they said the patients believed they had been helped, which seemed to make a difference in their perception (of the prognosis of their condition).

"This study has important policy implications," said lead investigator Dr. Nelda P. Wray, "We have shown that the entire driving force behind this billion dollar industry is the placebo effect."

Reports of this study in newspapers and online journals where invariably headed 'Knee Surgery Proves No Better Than Placebo' when they could have just as easily been headed 'Placebo Knee Operation Proves More Effective Than Real Surgery' or even 'Power Of The Mind Proves More Effective Than Surgery!'

The writers of the newspaper and internet reports also concluded that the study indicated that osteoarthritis knee surgery was ineffective and unnecessary and that hospitals should stop performing the operation; placebo operations not being a practical or ethical alternative practice. This conclusion is of no benefit to patients who are suffering from the condition, unless some steps are made to help the patients create their own healing through the informed and practiced use of deliberate belief.

It is acknowledged that placebo is effective in pain relief. The study above indicates that the placebo initiated actual structural change and healing within the body. The placebo recipients experienced a long-term benefit from a painful and debilitation condition, just through believing that they had had surgery. Presumably healing had taken place within their knees that would otherwise not have happened. But is the placebo also effective in conditions that are perceived to be more serious or life threatening? Can the placebo effect cure cancer?

Consider that every new cancer drug that comes to market is extensively trailed against placebos to quantitatively prove that it is more effective than placebo alone. This is a very expensive and time consuming procedure which the drug companies are legally required to do.

To say that a drug is more affective than a placebo is to acknowledge that the placebo is effective to some extent. If placebos did not have a measurable effect at curing cancer (or, in fact, every ailment known to mankind) they would not be used as a yard-stick in every drug trial.

Drug companies know exactly how effective placebos are, but they routinely overlook and downplay the implications with the use of the label 'placebo effect'. The very use of the label obscures what is actually happening; patients in drug trials spontaneously create cures for cancer because they believe that they have been given a cancer drug.

The Ig Nobel Prize winning study cited above shows that the placebo effect is proportional to the patient's level of expectation of the effectiveness of the medicine. Given that volunteers in a trial know that they might be receiving an inert placebo and that even if they are receiving the real drug, it is experimental and unproven, then their level of expectation must be relatively low. The power of their belief is not fully engaged, yet still a measurable curative result is achieved.

19

Drug companies' challenge is to come up with a chemical compound that is measurably more effective than the placebo and bring it to market in a rush of fanfare and expectation before its effectiveness fades away. Cancer drugs are known to lose effectiveness over time; some patients fail to respond, expectation drops, the medicine looses the glamour of a new wonder drug, doctors stop prescribing it and it spirals down as its it looses the power of the placebo.

This suggests to me that the effectiveness of actual medicine is still mostly due to the placebo inherent in every medical interaction. The fact that a medicine is new, it's hard to get and that it's very expensive all add to the patient's expectation of a cure.

People cure themselves through belief; the drugs and medical procedures are a focus for the belief and can be assistive in a chemical sense or can be destructive. Until we develop the ability and faith to create belief in our own healing powers we will continue to be reliant on the magic of pharmaceuticals and high-tech medical procedures to convince us that we can overcome our diseases.

Defenders of the allopathic biomedical model use the placebo effect to explain away other modalities of healing, particularly in the case of Homeopathy. This is a cruel irony as science has no explanation for the placebo effect in the first place so it's hardly an explanation for any other healing phenomena.

That an inert substance given to a patient who believes it to be an appropriate and effective therapy will cause the patient to experience an improvement in their condition has no scientifically described mechanism. The cause and effect cannot be adequately linked, apart to say that, somehow, the patients' belief in the efficacy of the medicine must have a positive effect on their healing or experience of pain and other negative symptoms.

Interestingly, the power of the placebo is so strong that there are even cases of placebo side effects. A patient, for example, may receive a placebo as part of a clinical trial and consequently develop a rash.

Some medical doctors are beginning to study the placebo effect, and consequently the power of belief and suggestion, as a valid healing technique in its own right. If a patient can be fooled into creating self-healing through their belief in their doctor and his/her medications can they not be encouraged to recognise and employ the power of their belief directly?

Essentially, science has co-opted a non-scientific, naturally occurring phenomenon, i.e humankinds' ability to self-generate a healing through positive belief and expectation, and given it a veneer of scientific acceptance by labelling it as an effect.

The deceit involved in prescribing a placebo goes further than just denying a patient the truth about the identity of a pill; it denies the truth of the patients' ability to heal themselves.

If you can get well by taking a sugar pill then you don't need any drugs, you also don't need a sugar pill. What you need is faith in your ability to heal.

Lolette Kuby writes;

'I believe that the medicine of the future will concentrate on triggering placebo effects. Encouraging patients to have faith in their ability to cure themselves will produce more cures than are dreamed of in our present medical philosophy.'

The Nocebo effect is related to the placebo in that it is the negative therapeutic outcome that a patient experiences through negative expectation of either a treatment or a medication. It is the voodoo hex and black magic curse of the witchdoctor as well as the list of possible side effects on your medicine bottle. It is the serious look on the faces of your friends and family and the statistical evidence of mortality rates. It is the dire advertisements urging you to buy life insurance and medical insurance. Anything that leads you to create a negative belief about your future health is a nocebo.

I recently had a personal experience of nocebo. When I first started taking chemotherapy I quickly became very nauseous and vomited repeatedly. I had been prescribed with anti-nausea drugs by my oncologist but didn't take them until I was already sick and found them not very effective. The vomiting passed after the first day but the nausea stayed with me for the full 40 days of the course of the chemo even when my doctor tried me on a more powerful anti-nausea drug, Zofran. The course of chemo came to an end and my nausea gradually abated until I was feeling relatively normal, then came the time to take another 5 days of chemo, at twice the strength as previously. I had to go into town to collect the chemo from the chemist but I already had some Zofran so I thought to prepare my body by taking the anti-nausea drug before I get the chemo into my system. I took one Zofran pill and then set off to the chemist only to find that the order had been messed up and my chemo wasn't going to be in until the next day. The trouble was, my nausea was already kicking in, when all I had taken was one anti-nausea pill! I realised that due to my previous experience of feeling sick while taking the drug, I had associated the anti-nausea pill with the feeling of nausea and my belief (association and expectation) caused my body to respond with the old feeling. My belief was stronger than the drug! This was a very helpful discovery to make and has helped me control my nausea without the drug as my treatment has progressed. It is very interesting when you notice that a drug can be a facilitator of ease or disease depending on your expectation.

Being told you have a terminal disease is, in effect, a nocebo, and it can have a deleterious affect on your health in addition to the condition you are already experiencing. Being given a negative prognosis not only defines the reality that you are sick in the present moment but that you will get sicker in the future.

Many people have died in very short-order after receiving a terminal diagnosis and it's not unreasonable to assume that they were victims of the nocebo effect!

I was recently told the story of a lady who was given a two year life expectancy by her doctor and she went home and marked the date on her calendar; sure enough she died within a week of the projected date. I guess she saved herself from having to live with uncertainty but I wouldn't recommend this degree of obedience to a doctors' prediction.

My oncologist is obviously aware of the power of both the placebo and nocebo effects and tries conscientiously to say nothing that could be interpreted as negatively or over-positively predictive about my life expectancy. He has let the cat out of the bag once though when I told him that I was concerned about the long-term effects of having my brain irradiated. His somewhat incredulous reply gave me the impression that long term effects were the least of my worries and getting through the next two years was going to be a pretty good outcome for me!

If you have any negative expectations about your health or longevity, no matter how you came to have them, then you need to do something to reduce their power. Negative expectations lead to negative experiences just as positive expectations lead to cures. The first step is to recognise and own your negative expectations, and then you need to recognise that you decided to believe them in the first place. Even if you have a negative expectation because of a medical study, or because your doctor told you, or because of other factual evidence or experiences, you decided to believe the evidence and you are deciding to project that evidence into the future. Lastly you need to change your mind and believe something better. If you like evidence then look for new evidence that will help you create a positive expectation. If you can believe on faith then create faith. If you can imagine a better outcome then imagine a better outcome. Keep going until your expectations are positive and you can't imagine why you would entertain anything different; then you will be empowering the placebo effect rather than the nocebo effect.

Rigorous drug trials are designed double-blind; this means that neither the patient nor the researcher will know who is receiving the placebo and who is receiving the drug. This is so that the experiment allows for, and reduces, researcher expectation and bias which are known to have an effect on outcome. If the researcher knows they are giving you a placebo then this might influence the result you experience, or the results they record. This raises the question as to how much other peoples' beliefs can be a factor in your healing. Will your doctor's expectation that you only have a few weeks to live have any effect out your survival even if their belief is unexpressed? Will the beliefs of your friends and family have any impact on your experience? Will the beliefs and expectations of fellow sufferers influence you?

The question that you need to consider in the light of the power of the placebo, and especially the nocebo, is 'How susceptible am I to suggestion and the viewpoint of others?' You can get a feel for how susceptible you are by considering the following questions:

- Do I readily believe what I am told?
- Do I want others to believe the same things I do?
- Do I make up my own mind or let others make it up for me?

- Am I placing my faith in the abilities of my doctor, medical institutions, or the power of medications over the healing ability of my body?
- Can I create faith in the healing power of my body?
- Can I use the power of the placebo deliberately?

If you think that you are susceptible to the beliefs of others, and we all are to some extent, then there are three possible strategies you can adopt:

- You can try to control what others think. This is not a very satisfactory strategy as it's a lot of hard work and people do resist being controlled, but if you can be persuasive and manipulative enough then you might get others to hold the beliefs that you think will be beneficial to you. Strangely enough, a lot of people adopt this strategy as a regular practice! Advertising, education, government legislation and propaganda are all attempts to control or influence what others think.
- You can choose who you will let influence you. If your doctor has no belief in your survival then find another medical practitioner who honestly believes that you have a chance to live. If you are surrounded by people who are negative then associate with people who have faith; hang out with spiritual practitioners or people who have survived serious illness. Read survivor stories on the internet. Read positive books about healing. Immerse yourself in positive belief so that the evidence supports your certainty that you can heal. Meet people from the Unity Church. Talk to Avatar masters.
- You can develop your willpower and your belief in your own authority. Ultimately, other people can only influence you if you let them. Make decisions, choose to believe in yourself, learn to meditate, practice yoga or do the Avatar course, whatever it takes.

It's an interesting phenomenon of our society but we appear to be prepared to believe in, and ascribe power to, absolutely anything imaginable except our own creative power. The placebo and nocebo effects, which are involved in every healing instance, are testament to our awesome self-healing capacity that needs only to be believed in to become an experiential cure.

Questions to consider:

- How am I being influenced by nocebos (negative beliefs and expectations)?
- How can I avoid or mitigate these nocebo influences?
- How can I deliberately benefit from the placebo effect?
- How can I maximise my faith in my chosen treatment or therapist?
- How can I improve my belief in my body's ability to heal?
- What actions can I take based on an expectation of improving health?

Questions for caregivers and supporters to consider:

- Are my expectations of the patient's health and future supporting their recovery?
- Are my words and advice placebo or nocebo in effect?
- How can I encourage realistic positive expectation?

Chapter 4

Science is a Method

Modern science has been a voyage into the unknown, with a lesson in humility waiting at every stop. Many passengers would rather have stayed home.
Carl Sagan

Isn't science great?

Where would we be without the benefits of science?

From before birth to after death we are sustained and protected by the ingenious products of scientific enquiry. So it comes as a bit of a let-down when we are told that science can no longer help us. It can, in fact, feel like betrayal and abandonment when we are told, by a confirmed and respected medical scientist, that our condition is fatal or incurable.

Lets look a little closer at science.

Science is a methodology and it has rules, practices and procedures. For a study, theory or an observation to be considered scientific it must be shown to be based on these rules and then be accepted within the scientific community. Studies need to be rigorously designed, results statistically significant and experiments repeatable with consistent outcomes. Due to these practices science has grown into a cohesive body of knowledge that we generally trust to be true and valid. The scientific viewpoint is considered the peak of rational thinking and it has spawned a burgeoning technology that has changed most aspects of our lives and has greatly exacerbated our impact on the planet

Modern medical practice is firmly based on scientific rules and procedures. Your doctor is a scientist and his/her authority and expertise is based on years of training and experience and backed up by a significant body of acquired knowledge, professional organisations, research organisations, private international companies and government administrative bodies etc. So when a doctor makes a declaration that your condition is fatal or incurable it's as if the voice of science is nailing your coffin shut, when actually, the statement is totally unscientific and unproven.

In science it is impossible to prove anything. No experiment can prove anything because no matter how carefully the experiment is designed, no matter how big the survey size is, there is always the chance that a datum exists that will prove the experiment wrong but was not counted or included in the survey/experiment.

To scientifically prove that a disease is incurable the study would have to include every incidence of that disease that ever existed, exists presently or will exist in the future and show that no person has, or will, ever survive; which is obviously impossible. Science gets around this hurdle of not being able to prove anything by creating an alternative hypothesis, i.e that disease x is curable, and sets out to disprove this, which can be done statistically with a smaller sample size. Once the alternate hypothesis (the null hypothesis) is disproved the hypothesis is <u>assumed</u> to be true. The hypothesis that the disease is incurable then stands until it is proved wrong and a single incidence of someone surviving the disease is enough evidence to prove it wrong. The trouble is, when people do survive an incurable disease they are often not counted by medical science, for a number of reasons:

- Data is usually only considered scientific if it occurs within a formal scientific study.
- Personal affirmations of survival are considered unscientific and unverifiable.
- People who survive may do so after having left the care of their doctor and turned to an alternative modality of healing.
- People may have survived the condition without it ever having been diagnosed by a doctor or treated.
- When someone presents their evidence of surviving a terminal disease believers in the scientific paradigm would rather challenge the veracity of their evidence than consider changing a scientific fact.

As a sufferer of a condition all you need to do is find one example of someone who has survived your condition and you can then decide for yourself that it's not incurable.

So what a doctor can say, which would have more scientific rigour and honesty is, 'Medical science has failed to find a confirmed cure for your condition.' Even this statement is fudging the issue unless he/she adds, 'that I currently know of.'

It's hard to admit to personal ignorance, especially when you are considered an expert and people are putting their life in your hands. Maybe that is why some doctors will hide their ignorance behind the authority of a pseudo scientific declaration when faced with having to tell someone that they don't know how to help them heal.

Will this change of wording make any difference? I think so. The statements, 'Your condition is incurable' or 'You have only 3 months to live' are delivered as if based on scientific fact, they define a reality. The statement, 'I don't know how to treat your condition' is a declaration of personal truth, it doesn't need any backing up with facts or data, it just needs courage. The advantage of the second statement is that it allows for alternatives, it doesn't define a reality where the patient is expected to die. The patient is free to consider that spontaneous remission is a possibility or that alternative treatments are a possibility or that they will survive due to their will or the grace of God without making their doctor or science wrong.

Another curious aspect of science is that it is built on the premise that there is an ultimate objective reality and that scientific researchers can design their experiments to reveal this reality without interference from their subjective experience. Experiments are designed to rule out the expectations and beliefs of the researchers. Well, at least that is the ideal. Considering that every experiment is the product of the human mind and every scientific perception of the universe is a human mind perceiving, is it really possible to remove the subjective viewpoint? We pretend that science is describing the universe when it can only ever be describing our perception of the universe, and this might not be the same thing.

If you further consider that science is based on the premise that our beliefs about reality are not relevant to reality then science is at a bit of a loss when it comes to studying belief and the effects of consciousness. The idea that one's beliefs interact with an undefined all-that-is, to create a perceivable, measurable reality is anathema to the basis of the scientific method and throws everything into question.

How can science determine if belief creates reality without the beliefs of the researcher influencing the reality they discover?

Essentially, belief and science are different realms of consciousness and you can operate in one or the other. If science is predicting a dismal and short future for you then your recourse from science is belief.

The scientific method was initially formulated for the study of the physical world and it has been a very successful endeavour so far; our understanding and mastery of the physical sciences has led to our modern lives of wealth and ease.

The physical world lends itself to study. It is consistent in behaviour, across both time and space; gravity behaves consistently irrespective of location or time (on a human scale of measuring). Physical matter also seems unchanged by its interactions with the consciousness observing it; looking at a rock doesn't appear to have any effect on the rock (in contrast to consciousness which is not consistent in time and space and will change as soon as it is observed). It's this consistency of the behaviour of physical matter that allowed science to predict the behaviours of materials with reliable accuracy and to discount the presence of consciousness as being of importance.

Newtonian physics describes the motion of objects using mathematical formulae; it describes a view of the physical world operating like a vast machine with every movement and action predicated by precise and definable rules.

Human bodies are physical in nature and medical sciences developed with a mechanistic viewpoint. In the 17th century, when the methodology and scope of scientific enquiry were being formulated, Rene Descartes dismissed the idea that mind influences the physical character of the body. In his view, science was concerned with the behaviour of matter and the mind was not material in nature and consequently immeasurable and indefinable, (and best left as the concern of the Church). This dividing of mind from matter, which is still present in scientific thinking today, leads to the philosophical conundrum of how immaterial mind can be connected to a material body.

31

Can consciousness influence matter?

Everyday evidence of the physical world would suggest that it can't but as physics has progressed; looking at matter in ever finer detail, it has discovered that consciousness does influence matter at the sub-atomic level. The behaviour of sub-atomic particles can be changed purely by observation. If you find this hard to believe than I suggest that you have never tried cloud busting. Lie on your back and look at a cloud. Start with a fine wispy one, and stare at it intently with the intention of making it dissolve. With practice you will realise that you can dissolve clouds solely by observing them with intention (practice with small wispy ones rather than thunderclouds). I know because I can do it.

The human body is a solid creation of matter and, on a gross scale, it reacts in predictable ways according to the nature of that matter. The body is subject to gravity and will fall if unsupported. The body is subject to the laws of Newtonian physics and will react predictably to applied forces. But the human body is intimately inhabited by the spirit of the consciousness that identifies with it. Descartes considered this 'ghost within the machine' as impotent to effect the body, but is it?

The mere fact that we can deliberately move our arms and legs etc shows that the mind is connected to the physical matter of the body; somewhere there is a crossover from conscious thought to conscious movement – a non physical intention becomes a physical cascade of chemical reactions and the constriction of muscle fibres.

In his book *Biology of Belief,* cell biologist Bruce Lipton demonstrates that the 50 trillion cells in our body are equipped with receptors responsive to chemical messengers as well as receptors tuned to respond to vibrational energy fields. These receptor 'antennas' read energy fields such as light, sound and radio frequencies and can induce changes within the cell, such as activating genes within the cell's DNA. 'Biological behaviour can be controlled by invisible forces,' he writes, 'such as thought, as well as it can be controlled by physical molecules like penicillin, a fact that provides the scientific underpinning for pharmaceutical-free energy medicine.'

Pharmaceutical medicines effect the chemistry of the cells through interacting with the chemical receptors embedded within the cell membranes; they turn on or turn off chemical information systems already present within the cell. Lipton points out this process is energy expensive for the cell and is much slower and more inefficient than the information that can be transmitted through the 'energy' receptors. This suggests thought and belief (and tuned energy therapies) can have a greater effect on the chemistry and behaviour of the cells than chemical based therapies can achieve.

Deepak Chopra explores the crossover point where thought becomes a physically measurable (ie scientific) reality in his book *Quantum Healing*. These crossover points, he claims, occur within our cells at a molecular level where an innate intelligence operates.

> 'Our belief in our healing can trigger a cascade of physical healing responses within our body that are far more effective and intelligent than any that can be administered by a doctor.'

The placebo effect is an interesting anomaly or crossover between the two realms; medical science recognises the effect because it has to, even though it has no scientific basis. The placebo effect is a physical phenomena, i.e a change in the body, created by a non physical phenomenal, i.e a belief. The mind's expectation of pain-relief can trigger the 'energy' receptors on the cell membranes to produce the same effect as when the chemical receptors get triggered by molecules of analgesic medication.

If you decide on an alternative course of treatment or faith healing etc please be warned that well-meaning people who believe in the scientific paradigm will think it their duty to make you see reason. They will try to warn you that what you are embarking on has no scientific basis. They will say that it is not clinically proven and therefore you shouldn't put your faith in it. If you want to see an example of this behaviour visit www.quackbusters.com this site contains lists of alternate health practices and why doctors don't think they are effective. If this happens to you just remember you are not conducting a scientific experiment nor writing a scientific paper requiring peer review; you are fighting for your life!

The scientific viewpoint, based on clinical studies and statistical analysis has already proven that people like you and I are going to die of our ailments. This is why we need to look beyond the restrictive blinkers of scientific sight. Science is about what has been, we are about creating a positive future for ourselves. The treatment, or non-treatment, that you choose can work for you even if it is not clinically proven, it's up to you and the power of your belief.

Questions to consider:

- Is my faith in science currently helping me?
- How relevant is scientific theory to my personal experience?
- Will my recovery prove anybody wrong?
- What matters more; being right or changing my beliefs?
- What beliefs am I prepared to give up to experience healing?
- Can I only trust something if it is proven?
- What evidence do I need to believe in something?
- Are there any real, incontrovertible, facts in medicine?
- Is scientific truth the only truth?
- What do I believe?

Chapter 5

Some viewpoints on Statistics

There are three kinds of lies: lies, damned lies, and statistics.
Benjamin Disraeli

Statistics are useful tools, especially if you are dealing with populations or multiple events. Statistics are useful only when you don't know stuff. There's little value in knowing the statistical probability of something that has already happened; the outcome is certain. Statistics are a handy tool when you are uncertain, they can predict possible outcomes and allow you to make plans to cover the most likely.

Statistics do have inbuilt limitations though; they are absolutely useless at predicting a singular event in space and time if it has never happened before. If something hasn't happened before then there is no data to make predictions on.

Are you a singular event in space and time or have you happened before? Has this health challenge happened to you many times before and were the outcomes recorded and measured? I doubt it.

Statisticians rely on assumptions. They assume that rep-eatable behaviour, of things or people, indicates some unchanging reality. They assume that the future outcomes of events or processes will follow the same course as the outcomes of previous, similar events or processes which have been accurately measured and recorded.

But you are unique in space and time. Did the clinical study that yielded the data, that generated the statistics, which predict your imminent death, include a Spanish speaking cross-dresser who plays the oboe, or a '............ (define yourself here).............'? Count yourself out of the study and the statistics don't apply to you. You have never been measured.

Most clinical studies are based on a selection of people whose common denominator is that they are suffering from a specific disease and receive a specific treatment within a controlled environment. The experiment is really only to assess the effectiveness of the treatment; it's not about the subjects, their beliefs, expectations or experiences. The study will be designed to reduce or remove uncontrollable variables. So are you a study subject within a controlled environment? Do you want to become a dot on the graph? No! Then see yourself as an uncontrolled variable and count yourself out of the data.

Statistics are all based on past data being used to predict future events, but things change. You can change. You can change your mind or your intention or the course of your life. You are new data which is not contained within the study and probably won't be counted. So if the statistics aren't going to pay any attention to you why pay attention to them?

The chance of tossing a coin and it landing on heads is 0.5 or you could say the occurrence of getting heads is 50%, but this only becomes apparent if you toss the coin many times. With multiple tosses you get the occurrence of heads coming close to 50%. The more tosses, the more predictable the outcome.

How many times are you going to experience this event of living or dying within this lifetime? Only once right? You are either going to experience a 100% recovery or 100% death. You are an individual, not a population, so statistics don't apply to you.

Doctors and medical authorities deal with populations; they roll the fatality dice many times so they experience death by disease as a statistical event. Doctors, with the best intentions, give advice based on statistical evidence. If the statistical evidence for a certain disease was 10% survival then the doctor could tell 9 patients they are going to die and one they are going to live and that would more accurately reflect the actual outcome; there's not going to be 10 patients 10% alive. A doctor can't do this though so they give everybody the same chance, based on the disease information and their own judgement.

Even if the statistical data is accurate and relevant to your experience, you can live a lot longer than the mean survival prediction without defying statistics.

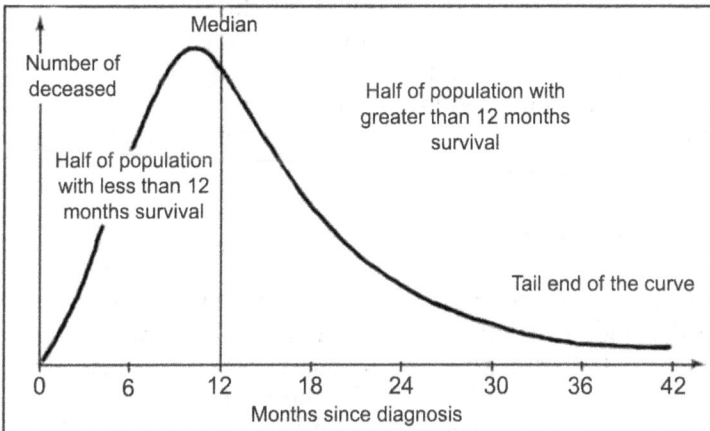

This graph is a typical cancer survival curve depicting a median survival of 12 months which means 50% of population will die before 12 months and 50% after. The height of the curve indicates the number of deceased and it peaks just before the median mark. From a purely chance perspective, the probability of dying increases over time until just before the median is reached and then drops quite steeply after the median. Notice the tail end of the curve begins to level off and can extend for a very long way, indicating some people can live a very long time; many months and years past the median survival rate. If you have been given a median survival rate it doesn't mean you will die when you get to the median mark; the graph indicates once you reach the median then your chances of survival increase every day. The further you get past the median survival rate, the shallower the curve and therefore the higher the chances of survival. You just need to believe yourself to be one of the survivors and do what you believe is necessary to place yourself in the long tail of the survival curve.

If the statistical information is accurate, up to date and relevant, then the deaths within the disease population will respond within the predicted curve, however, there is no statistical data that can accurately predict where you, as an individual within that population, will be placed along the line of the curve. Dying at 4 months and still being alive at 28 months are both possible outcomes allowable within the statistical prediction curve, but as experiential realities, they are vastly different!

By the rules of chance, previous occurrences do not affect the outcome of a particular event, even when the statistics are fully known. For example you can toss a coin 8 times and get 8 heads and the chance of getting a head next time is unaffected, it's still 50%. Even if you have just tossed 60 heads in a row, which is very unlikely, the chance of the next toss being a head is unchanged. Each toss is a new event. So even if the last 300 people who had your disease died within 3 months it doesn't mean you will, and the factors involved in your survival are much more complex than the tossing of a coin, possibly beyond our ability to measure and predict.

So if you already know (by choosing to believe a statistic) one in four people who have your disease survive, and you find yourself eyeing up your fellow sufferers at your support group and wondering which three are going to die for you to survive, don't bother, what happens to the others will have no influence on what happens to you (unless you let it).

Considering the power of the nocebo, it's quite likely that a negative statistical prediction of life expectance will become a self fulfilling prophesy. Do the statistics predict a 10% survival rate because 10% survive or do 10% survive because they are told they have a 10% statistical chance of surviving?

Another viewpoint worth considering is that just about every statistic or clinical report you can access is probably already out of date. Clinical procedures and drug therapy regimes are changing rapidly and mortality rate studies take a long time to compile. By the time population studies are published the advances and changes in medical practices and treatment options are likely to make them no longer valid. For example; the statistical data from a 5 year study can only show what your chances of death/recovery were if you were diagnosed 5 years ago.

So it seems you are free to decide the outcome of your life; any prediction you make has got to be more accurate and appropriate than that of a statistician who has never met you, won't ever meet you and doesn't give a monkey's ass whether you live or die.

In summary:

- Statistics apply to populations not individuals.
- You are different to the study subjects so can experience a different outcome.
- Statistics assume an unchanging world, but things change.
- Statistics can be self-fulfilling prophesies and nocebos.
- You are a unique event is space and time.
- You can choose not to believe statistics.

Questions to consider:

- Are the statistics that predict my demise current, relevant and accurate?
- Do I have to believe what my doctor says?
- Can I find statistical data that supports a more positive outcome?
- Can I realise myself as being more source than the statistics? (ie can I believe in myself in spite of contradictory exterior data)
- How can I free myself from a nocebo statistic?

Chapter 6

Denial and Resistance

All inner resistance is experienced as negativity in one form or another.
Eckhart Tolle

Denial is pretending something doesn't exist, resisting is pretending it's not your responsibility.

Denial is something all 'terminal' patients have to deal with but what is it and how do we know when we are in it?

The oxford English dictionary defines three meanings for denial:

1. To declare a statement to be untrue.
2. To refuse to give or allow.
3. To refuse to acknowledge.

In terms of deliberately managing your beliefs about your disease, these first two definitions could be seen as being helpful: If you decide the statement 'your disease is incurable' is untrue, is this a deliberate exercise of your right to choose or is it delusional? Likewise with the second definition, if you refuse to allow the progression of your disease. This could be a deliberate act of an aware individual.

I think the clincher is in the third definition where one refuses to acknowledge. This definition implies the situation one is refusing is already present and real to you. You can't refuse to acknowledge something that doesn't exist in the first place. At some level we accept that we do have a potentially fatal disease but we use denial, a trick of the mind, to insulate our consciousness from experiencing the reality fully.

Denial is such a common and natural response to bad news that we must believe it serves us. Maybe we believe if we deny something then it will go away and we won't have to deal with it. Perhaps this is an effective strategy in the short term but sooner or later we do have to accept what we believe to be the reality of our situation and choose to deal with it.

The solution is to accept what <u>we believe</u> to be the reality of our experience rather than accept what others believe to be the reality or that there is an ultimate factual reality we have to conform to.

Our loved ones, our doctors and our friends will all have their concepts of the reality we should be accepting and they may well accuse us of being in denial if we refuse to recognise or acknowledge their version of reality. But denial is about what is going on in your universe, not theirs. It is perfectly valid for you to define your condition however you want to. Denial is only happening when you are denying what you really think is true.

Throughout the disease process you might find yourself going into denial many times as your mind attempts to deal with each new, and often unpleasant, symptom or dis-ability. You might even find yourself going into denial on receipt of good news; it's not uncommon for people to deny the reality of going into remission.

If you feel you might be in denial, a question you could ask yourself is; 'am I present and feeling the full extent of my situation?' If you are predominantly in your mind (thoughts, rationalisations etc) or feel distanced or unattached from your situation then you could well be in denial.

I recently had an experience of denial when I found I was unable to contact my oncologist for over a week. I had rung to cancel an appointment and was due to be starting a monthly round of chemotherapy the following week. The purpose of the appointment was so the doctor could catch up with me, check my blood stats and prescribe the chemo drugs. I, however, didn't want to make the 5 hour trip and considered the visit an unnecessary inconvenience and was trying to get him to make the prescription over the phone. So I had missed my appointment but didn't have a prescription for my drugs but felt totally fine and relaxed about the whole thing.

When my wife suggested perhaps I was a little bit in denial I told her it was her anxiety that she was experiencing and that I had no worries about getting my drugs in time. So she asked me 'what would someone have to believe in order to experience not being able to talk to their doctor?' (This phrasing is the start of an Avatar exercise called transparent beliefs from the book, *ReSurfacing®: Techniques for Exploring Consciousness* by Harry Palmer). I answered the question, and Stephanie kept repeating it until I had a realisation (became aware of the feeling) of what I was denying. I had been pretending to myself I wasn't sick but I really believed I was. I just wanted to be living a normal life and was using denial to trick myself. The clue that I was in denial was the detached and casual way I was acting about something potentially important.

The solution to denial is to willingly acknowledge and admit what you believe to be true and what you believe to be real, not what you would like to be real. You can only give your full attention and creative power to creating the reality you would like to be real once you have acknowledged where you are truly at, otherwise your positive words and thoughts will be undermined by your unrecognised and un-owned fears. If you remain in denial your spoken words will sound false to others and you will lose trust in your ability to steer your own course. So, as my daughter's soccer coach says; 'dig deep' and honestly admit what it is you don't want to recognise. Maybe it's the fear of dying, of suffering or of having an incurable disease. Being honest with yourself and others is a crucial step to healing. Sure it might feel scary and it might feel like going backwards but being real about what you believe is a necessary doorway to self-respect and faith.

Resistance is trying not to feel or not accept something that is already happening. If you are resisting the idea you have a disease yet you are experiencing symptoms of the disease then you are in for a struggle. The reason why resistance is futile is because if you are resisting a disease then you are resisting an aspect of your body, which is an aspect of yourself. Try to fight and struggle against yourself and all you will experience is suffering, frustration and exhaustion.

Medical science leads us to believe a disease is an invasion; something is attacking us and it's therefore only sensible, from this viewpoint, to fight back. But this viewpoint is a denial of ownership and responsibility for the disease; it views us as victims. We rail against our fate and vow to fight to the death but all we are fighting is ourselves. A tumor is a growth of our cells. A heart condition is still our heart. A degenerative disease is our body degenerating and an infection is an expression of a weakness of our immune system. If we go to war with our diseases we are going to war with our body, when what our body needs is an ally.

When you have a disease some of your creative energy is already manifest in that disease, when you choose to resist the disease you are directing your energy against your energy. This is the theory behind the saying 'what you resist persists'. Resisted illness persists because you are unconsciously sustaining it with your creating energy and fixing it in place by your resistance energy, your energies balances out and the condition remains; at arms length.

Have you ever successfully resisted stress, a headache or pain through force of will? If you ever have managed it, I bet that as soon as you relaxed, the condition came back, probably with more intensity. Resisting stress adds stress to an already stressful situation. The way out of this situation is to relax and experience what already exists. Give-in to the pain. Surrender to your disease and allow yourself to experience the intolerable. You have a medical condition, it is causing you pain and threatening your life, so be it. Courageous acceptance of what is will bring you relief and peace; it will also give you a firm foundation from which to move forward. If you try to create healing over denied or resisted experiences and beliefs through heroic struggle, you might gain some success but as soon as you relax it will all come rushing back.

You can tell if you are resisting by noticing if you feel anger or frustration, if you want to complain and fight and blame, if your mind is agitated and you are thinking compulsively or if you feel you are under attack.

Resistance manifests as a familiar feeling or response which you will recognise as a pattern in your life; sometimes it can be tiredness or it can be a desire to eat, drink or smoke. Some people experiencing resistance want to argue or figure things out, they retreat from feeling and take refuge in theory, others go into a controlling or managing mode and get too organised to stop and really feel what is going on. Resistance can also manifest as a physical sensation. A few years ago our house burnt to the ground. Stephanie and I and the children naturally were distressed by this and we experienced a lot of grief and suffering. Stephanie experienced her resistance as a physical lassitude; she couldn't bring herself to walk up the path to the remains of the house as her legs felt too heavy and unresponsive to even take a step.

However it manifests, resistance is an effort to keep some perception or feeling at a distance, so it just takes a deliberate willingness to relax and experience what is there for you to experience.

Once you give-in and stop resisting, there could be discomfort, pain, grief, sadness or a feeling of powerlessness but these will pass as you willingly experience them. You might also experience insight into the cause of the disease and/or see a path to healing. Surrender brings a calm relaxed awareness and realisation. From this space you can choose to give up your burdens and move towards belief and faith.

Questions to consider:

- Am I in denial?
- What aspect of my illness am I denying?
- Can I acknowledge and accept the reality of my current experience?
- How do I usually experience resistance?
- What am I struggling against?
- What feelings do I not want to feel?
- What secrets am I keeping?
- What fears am I trying to hide from others/myself?
- Can I love and accept my body just as it is today?

Chapter 7

Fear

The only thing to fear is fear itself.
Franklin D. Roosevelt

What are you afraid of?

Having a serious disease is enough to make anyone scared and it's perfectly normal and expected to feel fear but we need to handle our fears and move on. The trouble with fear is that it attracts the very experience we are afraid of. When you put your attention on something it grows. The more attention you pay to your fears the more real they will become, and if you are already feeling anxious then this realisation can lead to even more anxiety.

Fear robs us of sleep, uses up our creative energy and interferes with our enjoyment of the present moment. Fear discourages us from being all we can be. Fear keeps us small.

Some of us feel fear acutely and some of us keep it suppressed, but we all experience it somehow. Sometimes fear manifests as abject terror but it can also visit us as anxiety and worry, or just a feeling of unease and uncertainty or an unwillingness to give something a go.

If you resist or deny fear it comes in the back door as irritability, anger or depression and if you try to avoid fear your life becomes small and restricted.

If you have a terminal disease then you will know fear, it has already visited you and will probably come again. You and I don't have the luxury of resisting or ignoring our fear, we need to face it. Harry Palmer, author of the Avatar materials says; 'Fear is a belief in your inadequacy to deal with something'. We have things we need to deal with so let's go looking for our beliefs about inadequacy.

List your fears; include the things you find yourself worrying about or have worried about in the past and the things you are avoiding thinking about. Go ahead and get it all out on paper.

Example, Fear:

I am scared of having a tumor reoccurrence and losing my ability to speak or care for myself.

Now take each subject on your list and write all the reasons why you think you are inadequate to deal with them. Try to get at least three beliefs for each fear but don't feel you have to stop there.

Example, Beliefs:

I will be made less if I can't talk (I will be dumb!)

Now for each belief review your past and look for evidence for holding this belief. Why do you believe this? What evidence do you have that you can't handle it?

Example, Evidence:

At times I have been hard to understand and people have ignored or discounted me.

As you do this process, allow yourself to acknowledge your fears, your perceived inadequacies and all the things that have happened in the past. Feel all the feelings connected with your fears and let yourself feel the beliefs.

Now, let's move on and create something better. Make a list of all the times you have overcome fear in the past; all the times you were courageous and did something you didn't think you would be able to do.

Example; Courageous act:

I agreed to have brain surgery to remove my tumor.

For each courageous act write at least three beliefs this action could exemplify.

Example, Beliefs:

I believe I heal well

Now review your life for all the evidence which support these beliefs.

Example, Evidence:

I never get sick and always heal easily.

Allow yourself to acknowledge all the times you have overcome your fears. Let yourself feel what it feels like when you take on something you are not sure you can do and succeed. Appreciate how much evidence you have that you are a courageous person able to handle everything the world throws at you.

Anchoring is a technique that helps you reconnect with a feeling. It involves remembering and feeling a specific time when you felt good and repeating a body action, e.g. clenching a fist, until the feeling and the action are connected in your mind. As you go over the times when you acted courageously, let yourself feel all the positive feelings and repeat a simple body action until your mind makes the connection and you can recreate the courageous feeling at will. Then, when you find yourself experiencing fear about the future, if you worry or fret or think you won't manage something, repeat the body action and you will be able to access the feeling of courage and success. Every time you get through your fear and achieve success, repeat the body action again, the anchor will grow stronger and fears will become a thing of the past.

Some questions to consider:

- How does my fear influence my experience?
- Will my worrying give me one more minute on this earth?
- What does fear create?
- What fears can I willingly reveal?
- What is there on this earth that can hurt my spirit?
- Can any physical disease overcome love or compassion?

Chapter 8

Do You Want to Live?

If you live to be one hundred, you've got it made. Very few people die past
that age.
George Burns

'Do you want to live?' is the question every healer has to ask their patients and 'Do I want to live?' is a question you need to ask yourself. Over and over again.

Why?

You might have wanted to live this morning but do you still want to live now; now that the pain is coming on, you feel nauseous and the hopelessness is back. It's your intention, moment by moment, that leads to the future you will experience out of all possible futures.

There are lots of books in popular culture which suggest that if you want something intently enough, write some affirmations or put a picture of it on your mirror, the universe (or God, great spirit, etc) will bring it to you.

Perhaps this will work but you have to put the effort in, you have to really believe. You can't trick God or the Universe. You are part of God (or the Universe etc) and what you experience as your life is you (a tiny small part) interacting with the rest, the big part. If your intention is not consistent and firm in your space how will it manifest in the Universe? Wanting to be alive, most of the time, or with most of your intention, could result in being dead some of the time or being only partially alive. (feel familiar?)

In *Love, Medicine and Miracles* Bernie Siegel, M.D writes;

> 'About 15 to 20 percent of all patients unconsciously, or even consciously, wish to die....In the middle of the spectrum of patients is the majority, about 60 to 70 percent. They are like actors auditioning for a part. They are performing to satisfy the physician.... At the other extreme are the 15 to 20 percent who are exceptional. They are not auditioning; they are being themselves. They refuse to play the victim.'

If you decide to die that's your choice and I honour it. When it comes the time I hope I can make the decision from choice. Not from hopelessness or fear or obedience or resistance but from choice.

Victor Frankle, who survived a Nazi concentration camp, writes;

> 'Everything can be taken from a man but the last of the human freedoms: his ability to choose his attitude in the face of any circumstances.'

Assuming you want to live, let us ask the question: how much do you want to live?' Bernie Siegel's measure of the exceptional patient is one who answers the question. 'Do you want to live to be a 100?' with a spontaneous and unconsidered 'Yes'.

Is that you? Do you want to live to be a 100 or would you like to define some conditions before making a commitment?

If you have manifested a potentially fatal disease I suggest to you that you don't actually, completely, want to live.

Lets work back from what you are experiencing; a life threatening disease – and explore the beliefs you hold which might have created it. What intentions have you been holding to bring this into being?

Does this attitude bother you? Am I going too far suggesting you might be responsible for creating this horrible condition which is ruining your health and threatening your life? Can you feel your resistance and indignation rising? Well just how do you want to see yourself?

Do you see yourself as a victim? There's plenty who will support you in this role. The biomedical model of health sees the body as a machine (the doctor is the mechanic and you are just the hapless owner). Machines breakdown, bad luck, you got sick, not your fault! This attitude lets you off the hook but where can you go with it? The trouble with not taking any responsibility is that it doesn't give you the ability to respond (response-ability).

So maybe you didn't keep up with the maintenance or misused the structure or put the wrong fuel in. Taking a bit of responsibility will help you here.

More about the victim viewpoint later.

If you believe that life, death and disease are just chance events then there's little you can do about any of it and you will find yourself the victim of statistics and you already know the statistics. Do you really want to believe this, considering the position you are in?

You could see your fate as being decreed by outside sources: doctors, the cancer, the stars, God. Then supplication, hope and acceptance are your only options.

You could see yourself as a spiritual being learning about life. In this case your brush with mortality is a lesson: wake up, pay attention! What is your higher-self trying to tell you? Try to see yourself as the creator of your life. You didn't deliberately and consciously bring this healing crisis into your life, but here it is. Assume responsibility for it and then experience your way through it.

Look for the beliefs and intentions you hold which might have brought your illness into being and accept responsibility for them.

- Have you smoked or taken drugs?
- Do you drink too much?
- Do you overeat?
- Did you overwork?
- Did you pass by on opportunities to love, to be loved?
- Do you harbour grievances?
- Is there something on your conscience you need to confess?
- Have you failed to follow your intuitive guidance?
- Have you made less of your life than you could?
- Do you make less of others?
- Do you harbour hate, envy or bigotry?
- Are there members of your family whom you are estranged from?
- Are you not at peace with yourself?
- Do you live with fear and anxiety?
- Do you avoid chances to give help or charity to others?
- Do you beat yourself up?
- Do you resist change?

Make your own list...

This list could be endless but if you want to change the experiences you are attracting then you need to find what beliefs are motivating your creations, experience your way through them and start believing something different.

Ok so I am an Avatar Master and Avatar teaches personal responsibility, so I have had to walk my talk. Yes I confess I have not been living my life as though I wanted to live to be a 100! I can say yes to most, if not all, of the counter intentions listed above. (I call them counter intentions as they are actions based on beliefs and intentions which are not motivated by love of life, self or others)

Recently, on an Avatar course, I discovered I had, at some time, decided I would never feel divine love, or even unconditional love, while I was in this body on this planet, so my yearning for union was leading me towards death. This is a very common type of belief for a cancer sufferer and I need to fully integrate this belief as part of my healing. I will know when that is done when I can feel and experience divine, unconditional love for myself and others.

Every thought, intention or compulsive reaction you experience has been created by you and carries with it a portion of your creative energy. You need that energy now if you really want to live.

Questions to consider:

- How much do I want to live?
- Are my actions the actions of someone who desires to live fully?
- What am I prepared to give-up in order to live?
- What am I prepared to do in order to live?
- What am I prepared to change in order to live?

Chapter 9

Reasons to Live

*Stuff your eyes with wonder . . . live as if you'd drop dead in ten seconds.
See the world. It's more fantastic than any dream made or paid for in
factories.*
Ray Bradbury

Anybody who works in a hospital will know that lots of people die just after Christmas. This could be attributed to the eating of too much chocolate and other rich foods or to the inevitable stress of the festive season but that's not the case.

The majority of the people who die just after Christmas do so because they believed they were dying and had made an effort to 'hang on until Christmas'. I know of one cancer sufferer who is currently hanging on for his fourth Christmas since his diagnosis. "We have already had three Christmases that we thought would be our last," he says, "so we made them big ones, for the kids' sake."

Since starting on this writing project I have heard so many stories of people who kept themselves alive long past medical expectation because they had a rock-solid reason to live. Craig Butler, an Avatar Master told me this story about his mother Willa.

'My mum died from cancer when I was 23. She was diagnosed with terminal illness when I was 10 and she decided she wasn't going to let what a doctor told her get in her way of doing what she felt was her mission in this life. Her primary aim was to support my brother and me to be successful in our lives and she achieved that. She survived all the way until I graduated from university and my brother completed his exams to be a master plumber, before she passed on, so 13 years extra. Along the way she supported her friends and extended family to be successful in whatever they decided they wanted to be. The reverend at her funeral told the congregation he felt more inspired by her than he could give back in return when he was ministering to her in the last few months of her illness.'

Some people hang on until their birthday or until their children graduate or even, until they prove their doctor wrong.

It doesn't really matter what your reason for living is; as long as it inspires you and engages your will. A specific event in time is a good goal to aim for as long as you make another goal when you get there or are satisfied to die once it is reached.

I have come up with a number of my own reasons to live which stretch into the future:

- I intend to be well for my next Avatar course in one month's time.
- I am going to be well to go on holiday with Stephanie in October.
- I am going to live to benefit from my free Wizard's course review in Florida in February. (I'd hate to die with unused credit, I'm Scottish after all).
- I am going to go to Bali next year and Nepal the year after.
- I am going to live long enough to see my daughters graduate from school and college.
- I am going to live long enough to prove this book right. (I know that my living isn't going to prove me right, just like

my dying isn't gong to prove me wrong; but I'll think I'm right and I like that!)

I'm sure I will make up plenty more reasons as I go along.

Reasons can be petty or they can be noble aspirations for the betterment of others and society in general. The main criterion of a good reason for living is that you really want to achieve it and it inspires you. The bigger and more exciting the reason then the more power it has to sustain you, (because it's the power you put into it).

So go ahead and make up some reasons to live.

- What would make your life worth living?
- What would inspire you to push through this suffering?
- What do you not want to miss out on?
- What do you still have to contribute?
- Is there a masterpiece you need to finish or to start?
- How much more loving do you want to get done?
- What would you like to set right before you die?

Seeing as you have recently had an unpleasant reminder that this lifetime is limited and the end might be sooner than you thought, now would be a good time to really consider what your life is all about. Just what are you here for? What has been the intention of your life and is it now enough to sustain you? Are you alive just to gather material possessions and be comfortable or what?

You will sometime die and lose everything you have strived for, but, unlike those who die suddenly, you have been graced with a warning and a time to prepare. How do you want to use this time?

Once you have decided on your reasons you need to invest in them. Direct your attention towards reaching your goals. Feel what it will feel like as your future goals are achieved and you are in good health to enjoy them. Spend time visualising the event in detail: If your goal is to make it to Christmas, who will be there? See their smiling faces in your mind' Imagine how happy you will be to have your family gathered around. Imagine the sights, the sounds and the smell of this future event – engage all your senses.

This is time well spent. Even if you end up dying and don't make it to your goal, at least you have taken your attention off yourself and your troubles for a few minutes. How refreshing was that? If you are going to be spending time thinking about the future then putting your attention on what you want to experience has got to be better than putting it on what you don't want to experience.

Isn't it funny how we can spend so much time visualising (worrying about) what we don't want to happen? Do you know of anybody who compulsively thinks of positive outcomes? Pollyanna was a fictional character who saw everything positively but to be labelled as a 'Pollyanna' is not usually complementary! I have heard of worrying being compared to going into a shop and looking at all the things you don't want, trying them on and then being surprised when you get them!

Healing is a present time activity, not something which happens in the future. Once you have your goal or goals you need to bring your attention back to the present moment. What do you need to do now that will be a step towards your goal, a step towards better health and a longer life? Is there a specific action you need to take; a health practitioner you need to contact, some health promoting exercises or an appointment you need to make? Is there a belief you could adopt that would help you? How much faith can you generate? Take action in the present moment.

Chapter 10

Victimology

Never be bullied into silence. Never allow yourself to be made a victim.
Accept no one's definition of your life; define yourself.
Harvey Fierstein

Modern Western society seems to be hell-bent on descending into a realm of victim consciousness. We have victims everywhere and institutions to support victims. The health systems and the legal systems thrive on the complaints of victims. Television dramas and news articles are all about victims. Support organisations support victims, laws protect victims, lawsuits reward victims and hospitals treat victims and so it goes on. Where are all these victims coming from?

Who is victimising all these people? Is there a class of people who are destined to become victims and another class of victimisers, but hang on, aren't the victimisers themselves just victims of bad upbringing, poverty or unjust social systems?

Within our current society you can blame anything except the victims and if you do start blaming the victims for their own sorry plight then you are probably very right-wing and possibly belong to a fundamentalist white supremacist organisation and are actually blaming victims for your own gain.

Of course I am getting a bit carried away here but it does sometimes seem we are surrounded by victims and we all, at times, experience being a victim. The question is, what do we do about it?

Blame, anger and retribution are possible responses, ones often modelled on TV and movies as entertainment, but are they a solution? Will they get you out of victimhood?

Since having cancer I have met a lot of other cancer sufferers, most of whom impressed me with their positive attitudes to their life with the disease, but there were some who were confirmed cancer victims. These people not only considered themselves victims of the disease but also of many other aspects of their current miserable existence; they felt they were not getting the support they should be getting from friends and family. They blamed their doctors for the wrong treatment they were getting. Their chemo schedules were getting mixed up through the incompetence of others. They were experiencing painful side effects of treatments and they focused their attention on their losses etc.

The trouble with seeing yourself as a victim is that there really is no way out of it. The best you can do is to convince someone else they are responsible for your troubles (ie blame them) but where does that get you? Victimhood doesn't evolve into something better. The more you focus your attention on being a victim the more alone and abused and powerless you will feel until you die, tragically bitter and defeated, by forces beyond your control. It's no way to live and it's no way to die.

Though there are some benefits to being a victim. Harry Palmer, author of the Avatar materials, lists these benefits of being a victim: (from The Forgiveness Option mini-course

- No expectation of responsibility
- The right to sympathy and pity
- No personal accountability

62

- Deserve to be supported
- Don't have to dress up
- The right to blame
- Not at fault
- Owed

How do we stop being victims? If our troubles stem from the actions of other people then the solution is forgiveness, we stop blaming the other and get on with our lives.

If your feelings of being a victim stem from your experience of illness then first look to see who you may be blaming (yourself? God? Your doctors? Manufacturers of carcinogens? McDonalds? Your parents?) Then begin the process of forgiving them, not for their sake but for yours.

Ask yourself

- Am I dying to prove anybody wrong?
- What will forgiveness cost me?
- What will I have to give up if I forgave person x, corporation y?
- What bastard will be proved right if I were to survive?

Of course, thinking that your dying will prove anything is just self-delusion. Maybe your ex-wife did make your life intolerable. Maybe you were treated as worthless by your employer and then abandoned when you got sick. Maybe your oncologist is an incompetent fool. But your death is not going to make the slightest difference to them. Forgiveness means giving up your position of being wronged and your judgments on the wrongdoers.

If you know how to forgive and have successfully done it before then now is the time to take an inventory of everyone you might be blaming and then forgive them as if your life depended on it, because it just might.

63

If you don't know how to forgive, or haven't managed to let go the resentment you feel for others then you could do with some help. Ask a friend or seek professional help --most religious teachers have experiential clarity on forgiveness. Better yet, seek an Avatar Master and/or download the Forgiveness Option Course from the Avatar website www.avatarepc.com

Harry Palmer also lists these benefits of forgiveness (from 'The Forgiveness Option mini-course')

- Accelerated Healing, both emotionally and physically
- Relief from stiffness and chronic pains
- Increase in physical strength
- Stress reduction
- Immune system booster
- Better digestion and bowel function
- More restful sleep
- Relief from depression and resentment
- Relief from self-sabotage
- More energy, more control (both physical and mental)
- Longer life
- More positive outlook
- Increased happiness
- Faster reaction time
- Friendlier, more tolerant
- More successful
- Increased awareness and intelligence
- Ability to establish new relationships
- Peace of mind
- A NEW LIFE

The cure to being a victim is to take responsibility. Bravely take a stand and declare, 'I am responsible for my life. I am responsible for the conditions of my life and for my actions and decisions. At times I am wrong and make mistakes but I take full responsibility for them. I have a life-threatening disease and I am responsible for my health, my attitude and whatever happens. I decide to live as best as I can for as long as I can!'

Taking responsibility is challenging but it will lead to growth and an increase in personal power, it could save your life.

Questions to consider:

- Are there times when I give-in to feeling like a victim?
- How does being a victim serve me?
- Who do I blame? God? My body? Myself?
- What can I take responsibility for in this moment?
- Who would I like to forgive?
- If I am going to die, how can I accept it?
- What do I need to do to be at peace with myself?

Chapter 11

Woundology and Identification with Disease

Every lesson is a widening and deepening of consciousness. It is a stretching of the mind beyond its conceptual limits and a stretching of the heart beyond its emotional boundaries. It is a bringing of unconscious material into consciousness, a healing of past wounds, and a discovery of new faith and trust.
Paul Ferinni

In the book, *Why People Don't Heal and How They Can* Caroline Myss explores the concept of woundology and explains how people can become so identified with their wounds they would rather suffer and die than give up their identity as victims and heal. Healing, especially for someone who has carried a lifetime of burdens and is strongly identified with their ailments will require them to open up to new experiences and to give up comfortable beliefs about their limitations and expectations.

Myss challenges us to get real about how we are using our wounds or our disease to our advantage.

What do you get out of being sick?

- Is there some feeling of righteousness you get through your condition?

- Do you make excuses for why you are not doing more positive things with your life?
- Do you compare your history of wounds with others?
- Do you compare your prognosis with that of others (my chance of survival is worse than your chance of survival)?
- Do you get off being responsible for working by being sick?
- Does your identity as a 'cancer sufferer' etc entitle you to special treatment or support?
- Would you lose the support of any special group (cancer support group, incest survivors, 12step groups etc) if you healed?
- Are you dependent on medical attention for any attention?
- Does your suffering earn you any respect? Does it make you noble?
- Are you bearing this burden for the sake of another?
- Do you feel your suffering benefits others in any respect?
- Does your suffering excuse you from being compassionate to others or let you off taking action to relieve the suffering of others?
- Does your suffering validate your anger, frustration or impatience with your loved-ones or caregivers.
- Do you withhold information about your illness to protect others?
- Do you ever exaggerate your symptoms or prognosis?
- Do you present yourself as stoic?
- Do you ever tell people you are fine when you feel like shit and want to cry?
- Do you take offence if people don't take consideration of your condition or treat you in a certain way?

If you answer yes to any of these questions then you could well be acting through an identity dependant on your illness (or on not being seen as being ill). If you answered no to all of them you are certainly acting through an identity and are in the grip of self-delusion.

These questions and others like them are ones you need to consider, not just once but moment by moment as you live through your illness and into health (or death); what identity am I creating now? When you allow an identity to form around your wounds, illness or suffering, that identity becomes part of your consciousness but acts like a little ego of its own, or an autonomous mental sub-program. It uses your creative energy to support itself. Any attempt you make to heal or to get real or to let go of old wounds will threaten this identity's survival and it will resist and act up.

Do you sometimes wonder where your negative thoughts and intentions come from, or why you just said something that was really negative and quite out of character? Do you sometimes say something and then feel it isn't quite true? Changes of viewpoint come about as you change your identities and this change can be subtle or extreme. People who suffer from bipolar disease flip between identities that are opposites in outlook and attitude and their whole personality and experience of life shifts radically as they do so.

Even healthy people have identities; they are how we create our personalities, and how we define ourselves to ourselves and others. Some identity is useful and a consistent identity helps people get comfortable with you.

The question you need to ask is, 'Is this particular identity serving me at this time and am I prepared to give up the ones that aren't serving me?' If you have defined yourself, or allowed another to define you, with identities such as 'a terminal cancer patient' or 'an incurable case' do you really want to keep them? Once you can recognise when you are identified with your disease you need to choose to stop feeding the identity with your attention energy. Any time you respond or act from an identity you make it stronger. If you find yourself wanting to impress someone with just how sick you are or indulge in feeling sorry for yourself, then you are acting through an identity and the identity is being sustained by the energy you could be using to heal.

Eckhart Tolle writes about identities in his book *The New Earth* (though he calls them 'painbodies'). He describes how they can lie dormant within the psyche but become activated in certain circumstances and then act to create drama that justifies and supports their viewpoint. An identity that is defined by the belief 'I deserve care because I am sick' will actively look for symptoms to justify its demands for attention. An identity defined by the belief 'I'm an abused woman' will see evidence of male abusive behaviour everywhere it looks. Identities can be cunning or persuasive or exhibit any aspect of character, to the exact extent that you can be cunning or persuasive etc because you think they are you. To disempower these painbodies or identities, says Tolle, you need to observe them as they arise within awareness, without judgement or reaction.

Other authorities would recommend meditation as a way of quietening the mind and bringing identities into awareness and thus integration. I would recommend the Avatar course as it teaches the deliberate creation and dis-creation of identities.

Why feed energy to a mental structure identified with being wounded and unwell when you could just as easily use that energy to create an identity defined as being healthy, happy and vigorous?

Questions to consider:

- How do I identify with my disease?
- What do I get out of identifying this way?
- What would I lose if I gave it up?

Chapter 12

Being Healthy and Healing

A healthy mind in a healthy body.
Hippocrates

What does this mean, being healthy? My understanding of the word 'healthy' is that it comes from the word 'hale' which means 'whole' and is reflected in the usage of the word wholesome. So to be healthy is to be whole.

Does being whole just refer to the body? Can you still be healthy with body parts missing? Yes you can. So the wholeness is referring to more than just the body.

Perhaps to be healthy is to be whole in body, mind and spirit, so it follows that to be unhealthy is to be less than whole in body, mind and spirit.

Perhaps your body has manifested a life-threatening disease to remind you that you are being less than whole in mind or spirit; some parts of your essential self are missing.

So if being unhealthy is about more than just the body, will treating only the body without addressing your spirit, soul or consciousness (however you understand your self) bring you back to wholeness?

- Can surgery or chemotherapy or any drug or remedy make you whole?
- Why did you get sick in the first place?
- Can your doctor make you whole?

Certainly doctors, drugs and therapy can stabilise your body and help it function better but they can't make you healthy; healing is a function of the mind and body.

To get back to wholeness you need to make it your intention to examine your consciousness with complete willingness and honesty and accept whatever you find as belonging to you.

I believe we depart from the state of wholeness through denial; we cut parts of ourselves off and deny ownership. For example, if you have ever said something like 'I am not selfish'—maybe someone is accusing you of behaving badly and although you do feel guilty it's the last thing you are going to admit, so you hurriedly bury or justify the evidence in your mind and protest your innocence. You are denying a part of your self and you become ever so slightly diminished. If you can allow yourself to acknowledge that in fact you are sometimes selfish, and allow yourself to feel the feelings you buried, then you are returning to wholeness.

Do any of us get through our childhood and schooling without becoming diminished? It seems unlikely. We come into this world with everything. We have the whole universe within us and no limits on our self-expression, no concept of guilt or appropriate behaviour or even the ability to perceive the existence of others. Is this what our parents wanted? No! They wanted a good boy or a good girl so the process of behaviour modification began. Some of us, the lucky ones with good parents, emerge in our late teens relatively functional and whole but some of us are so conditioned and pared down by our upbringing that we become just a tiny aspect of what we once were or could be. We are desperately trying to be a good boy or a good girl and resisting all those parts of ourselves that have been labelled 'unacceptable' by parents, authority figures or society in general.

- Can you get a feel for what aspects of your whole self you have suppressed?
- What are you too afraid to be?
- What particularly annoys you in other people: anger, greed, intolerance etc?
- What do your loved ones want from you that you feel you can't provide?
- What aspect of your self annoys your parents most?
- What would you never want to be?
- What makes you uncomfortable?
- Can you be OK with being wrong, with not knowing, with being at fault?

Welcome all the lost parts of yourself home, call your spirit back because you need to be whole to be healthy.

Given that there are many modes of healing and they all appear to work, for some people some of the time, and given the power of placebo and belief, what actually creates healing?

My conclusion is that healing is created by intention. One's intention to be healed sets off a train of events that leads to the experience of healing.

Intention motivates a period and an intensity of attention filtered through the belief structure of a healing modality. The success and rapidity of the healing depends on the intensity and clarity of the intention and the appropriateness of the actions taken.

It appears our bodies have a natural tendency to be healthy, we could think of this as a subconscious intention. Most

73

bodies, most of the time, are healthy and this state of health doesn't require any conscious attention from us to maintain itself. Small ailments, injuries, cuts, bruises, muscle strains and even broken bones will heal naturally. We come equipped with a powerful immune system which protects us from infections even though we are continuously exposed to infectious pathogens. This natural tendency gets overpowered when we stress the body or mind with injurious actions, intentions or beliefs. When we are experiencing disease we need to realign with our body's natural healing intention and empower it with our conscious healing intention. Our intentions are usually expressed through beliefs.

Beliefs define our reality but they also act as filters to the amount of attention we can successfully bring into the world. The more complex and structured the belief system the less attention we can channel through it. If you think of beliefs being filters on our perception you can get a feel for what I mean. If you are wearing red glasses everything you see will be red. If you are wearing red glasses and then also put on green glasses everything will get darker. The more glasses you wear the less you can see. Likewise the more beliefs you have to view the world through the less of the world you actually perceive. Taking belief filters off allows you to perceive more.

Training and education is often a process of taking on beliefs. Medical training is a very structured and intense indoctrination of beliefs. The biomedical model (allopathic medicine) is a complicated and rigorous belief structure. It has been developed over many years and has produced a very rigidly defined reality which we can perceive through scientific experimentation. Doctors who view reality through this belief structure can be very certain of the effectiveness of what they perceive, but they generally find it hard to perceive anything outside of the biomedical model or have the ability to focus much free attention on their patients: what they see is determined by their training! This is, of course, a generalisation and not intended as a disservice to the many compassionate and caring doctors who can see beyond their conditioning (training) and is meant as a comment on the institution rather than the individuals comprising it. It is also not a criticism; it's just the way the biomedical system works, the power is in the structure and the research and the doctor becomes the conduit to this power.

As a comparison, other healing modalities (Reiki, Avatar, Touch for Health etc) have a training process which requires the dropping of beliefs (thoughts, preconceptions, judgements etc) so the practitioner can perceive more subtle qualities of the patient and bring more, purer, attention to the practice, they become a direct conduit to a less defined healing power.

On a visit to a local general practitioner one would have an intention to experience a healing outcome, and the doctor is there with the intention of facilitating healing outcomes, so the intention is explicit. There is also the implicit healing intention in your body that seeks to return to a healthy state naturally. The doctor will give you some personal attention, often just a few minutes, and then usually prescribe a drug. In this case the period of attention is quite brief and can also be impersonal, in that medical doctors often have their attention focused on the disease and the appropriate remedial drug rather than on the patient as a whole. However, a drug is a form of artificial attention; it is pre-packaged and refined, like so many other things in our modern society. Attention has gone into the development of the drug and the testing and subsequent production and marketing. Through this process a strong belief has built up about the effectiveness of the drug for relieving a certain disease. When you go home from the chemists with your bottle of pills you are carrying a concentrated form of artificial attention, filtered and defined by the allopathic belief model with the intention it will cure you.

If you go to hospital to receive a course of radiotherapy for a cancer you will be strapped into a very expensive and highly technical machine which will bombard selected parts of your body with a mega dose of x-rays. This again is a concentrated and artificial form of attention given with the intention it will heal. During the process you will receive personal attention from the radiologists but mostly their attention is on their machine and the technical aspects of the treatment. There is a high degree of belief in the effectiveness of the method, otherwise why would anybody invest in a technique requiring 8 million dollar machines? You benefit from all the attention invested in the development of radiology, the investment in the training of the radiologists and in the building of the hospital as well as the certainty of the effectiveness of the treatment as proven by clinical studies: you don't need to supply much of your own belief to make it work.

If you go to a faith or energy healer, the infrastructure is often not as impressive. They don't have any expensive machinery or a huge hospital premises. They don't have clinical studies, or hugely complicated drug therapies. Often, all they bring to the healing is their own intention, their experience and training and an extended period of very personal attention. The attention you get is much more intense and focused and often for a longer duration than the attention you get from a MD. Also, their attention is filtered through a less dense belief structure, i.e a belief in magnetic healing or Reiki is less structured and restrictive than the biomedical model of medicine (again a generalisation, alternative healers can be judgmental, righteous or narrow-minded!).

Lolette Kuby, mentioned earlier, experienced a complete healing from cancer after a 5 minute revelation. She was reading Christian New Thought material with the intention of finding a healing and then had a vision where she received intense divine attention. I propose the attention she received, as it was not channelled through a human consciousness, (other than her own) was unfiltered by belief structures and very intense and pure which is why it created an instantaneous healing experience.

In Avatar practice we assist the students to integrate their beliefs and become more whole (ie healed) and free from suffering mainly by appreciating them with intense attention, as free as possible from any filtering beliefs (judgments, assessments, thoughts etc) and I have experienced many miracles through this process.

If you decide to manage your illness through meditation, belief management and visualisations or diet etc, you will need to supply most of the healing attention yourself and it will take a dedicated practice to achieve success.

In choosing your approach to your healing I advise you to honestly ask yourself how much healing attention you can personally manifest and sustain. If you have the dedication and will-power to manage your health through diet, meditation and visualisation then go for it, but if you know you are not so wilful and can be easily discouraged or distracted then choose a modality where you get healing attention through a healing practitioner or through physical or energetic sources (herbal remedies, drugs, energy therapies etc).

So the simplified recipe for healing is a two step process.

1. Create a strong and clear intention to be healed.
2. Manifest that intention by giving yourself, and/or receiving from others, sufficient appropriate attention filtered through the healing modality you choose to believe in.

Consequently the effectiveness and duration of the healing will depend on these variables.

1. How pure your healing intention is.
2. The strength of your belief.
3. The quality and duration of healing attention you can sustain or receive.

As an interesting corollary one can see that disease is also manifested by a similar process: first there is the intention to be unhealthy and then a period of actions or attention filtered through beliefs aligned with that intention. For example, take the case of a smoker dying from lung cancer. Given that just about everybody is aware of the dangers of smoking, one can only assume that people who continue to smoke have an intention which is not aligned with being healthy. Consistent attention to the intention in the form of action creates their ill health, i.e every time the smoker lights up they are reinforcing their decision to value momentary satisfaction over their long-term health. Their actions, motivated by negative intentions, overpower their body's natural healing tendency. They act through the belief filter 'I don't care about my health' and eventually create a life-threatening disease.

In my own case I discovered I had an intention not fully aligned with staying alive and experiencing the love I wanted to in this physical plane. Many times in the past when I have had the opportunity to be loving I have chosen, through fear or other limiting beliefs, to be less loving than I could have been. Now I realise that the cumulative effect of this attention filtered through negative beliefs has created the circumstances of my illness. The illness has, in return, brought me the opportunity to realise and integrate those beliefs and realign my intention to live and love with all my heart and soul. Once I readdress the imbalance my body will return to its natural tendency to be healthy.

Our illnesses come in a form that gives us clues as to how we have become unaligned in our intentions and also provides us with opportunities to heal, in the 'whole' sense of the word; they are signposts to what we need to integrate to become spiritually well.

With the hypothetical dying smoker I invented above, the belief that created their cancer was 'I don't care about my health' this belief allowed them to smoke for years and develop a disease. The disease gives them the opportunity to realise and reassess the belief; now that their life is threatened the belief 'I don't care about my health' becomes more apparent and important. If the belief is not recognised, owned and integrated then the continuing disease process will result in death. Reassessment of the belief is a crucial step in any healing process. They might still die if the disease is too far advanced, but at least they have the chance to address the underlying mental imbalance which created the physical disease.

As recipients of terminal diagnoses we may continue in our actions without changing our beliefs or intentions and we will suffer and die. If we are courageous and look at our beliefs and the intentions behind them, and take steps to change them, we may grow in wholeness and live.

If we want to address the question' why do people get sick' we will need to accept a very broad answer because there are billions of people in the world, millions of ways of being sick and many belief structures or models of disease to understand sickness through. To aid our understanding I will attempt a brief overview of the most common models of disease and explore how they answer the question of why people get sick.

Biomedical Medicine

The biomedical or allopathic model views the body from a material viewpoint; the mind is not considered as particularly relevant to sickness or healing. Because the medical model is underpinned and verified by scientific practise it is limited to only what can be measured and proven, this is also its greatest strength as well as a limitation. Because the body is viewed solely as a material object, sickness is seen as a physical process involving particles, chemicals, cells, organisms and organs etc. A disease is some physical fault within the structure or processes of the body and is treated in a physical way; with surgery, physical therapy, chemicals or radiant energies. This model works for many people and many ailments, and is especially effective for treating physical damage to the body, i.e accidents and injury and the physical degeneration of the body as exemplified by hip replacements and heart surgery etc.

The biomedical model fails to answer the question 'why do people get sick' because science doesn't concern itself with reasons or purpose, as that is the realm of mind or spirit and this has been outside the brief of science since the time of Rene Descartes. Science is concerned with 'how' rather than 'why' and the biomedical model is very good at determining how people get sick and its treatments are focused on either countering the symptoms or disrupting the mechanism of illness. One of the downfalls of this method is that people can experience a cure of a condition, but because the root cause has not been addressed, they might manifest the same condition again; I have read several books describing the stories of people who have survived up to four consecutive experiences of cancer, and I wonder why their bodies continue to manifest life –threatening diseases.

The best the biomedical model can do is to point to the physical causes of disease, i.e people get heart attacks because they have too much cholesterol in their blood. This begs the question, why do people have too much cholesterol? People have too much cholesterol because they eat fatty foods. Why do people eat fatty foods? Follow the physical cause and effect chain far enough and you come to personal choice; people choose to do things that are unhealthy through their knowing or unknowing adoption of beliefs.

One of the major achievements of the biomedical model is the germ theory of illness that demonstrates that all infectious diseases and sepsis of wounds is caused by microbes. Microbes can be seen through the microscope and the many effective treatments that have been developed to prevent their proliferation have saved millions from suffering and early death. It's a very effective theory and practice and vaccination programmes and antibiotics have made many infectious diseases a thing of the past within Western society. However there are some questions that the germ theory fails to answer, such as:

- Why do some people contract a germ borne disease when others don't, even when exposed to the germs?
- Why do microbes naturally present on the body sometimes become antagonistic to the body and cause disease?
- Why do plagues and outbreaks of infectious diseases manifest within specific populations at specific times?

The biomedical model is the official model of disease within Western culture in that it is the model that is practiced by state funded hospitals and promoted by medical authorities; it is protected by laws and financed by insurance companies. It is powerful and effective for creating curative treatments for many human ailments but there are consequences to believing in this model:

- It's very expensive and requires lots of technology. Some medications and treatments are so expensive that they are out of reach of many or the poorer people of the world or even of averagely well-off people within Western society if they don't have medical insurance.
- The focus of the biomedical model is primarily on disease rather than health. Much more money is spent on cure than prevention. A doctor's training involves many years of study of diseases and maybe a day's attention to what comprises a healthy person. One could say that the biomedical model is a sickness model rather than a health model.
- The biomedical model doesn't and can't explain why people get sick. Your personal experience of sickness is mostly explained by chance occurrence, population based statistics and precursor conditions.

- If you choose to avail yourself of this healing modality you become little more than a body; your consciousness and spirit become inconsequential in the therapeutic process and you have to rely on the judgments and beliefs of others.
- Practitioners and supporters of the biomedical model are generally antagonistic to alternative models of health; governments and insurance companies will not fund alternative treatments even though they may be much less expensive than biomedical treatments.

'Alternative' and Herbal Models of Healing

Many alternative models of healing are actually heavily based on the biomedical model in that they treat the physical properties of the patient and the disease but they prefer to use a herbal extract rather than a chemically produced drug to achieve the same result. The treatments are generally less expensive and therefore more accessible but the industry is less regulated and can be more easily taken advantage of by unscrupulous individuals who will sell cures which may be totally relying on the placebo effect. Belief in this model can be very effective if you find a reliable and knowledgeable practitioner but the negative consequences are that it still fosters reliance on an outside authority (the practitioner) and an outside source for the cure (the herbal medicine) and does not really address why people get sick or empower their ability to heal themselves.

One of the main beliefs within this model is that sickness is due to inadequate nutrition and thus many nutritional supplements are created to readdress this, e.g the belief that cancer is caused by a deficiency of amygdaline so taking this as a supplement is believed to prevent or cure cancer. It can be easily shown that scurvy is caused by a lack of vitamin C or rickets caused by a lack of vitamin D so most people can easily believe this health model but it fails to address why we have bad nutritional habits in the first place. What beliefs would cause people to adopt a diet that is obviously not health sustaining? Why will people consume fast-food and soft-drinks to the state of obesity or drink and smoke when they know it is killing them? Why have we created a world where many people are starving yet others are killing themselves by eating too much?

Mind-Body Medicine

Mind-body medicine is a recent offshoot from the biomedical model as individual doctors and therapists have begun to consider that the thoughts and beliefs of the patient are an integral part of their being and therefore needs to be attended to in any healing interaction. Notably, one of the best known pioneers of the mind body approach is Deepak Chopra. Dr. Chopra trained as a medical endocrinologist i.e trained within the biomedical model but because of his Indian origins he had access to Aruevedic medicine which doesn't suffer from the Cartesian divide between mind and body and incorporates mental and spiritual treatments within its practice. Mind-body medicine is really in its infancy at the present moment and as it develops I am sure it will address the question of why people get sick as it more fully explores the role of mind and belief in illness.

The Exorcism Model of Healing

In some cultures illness is seen as being an effect of demons. People get sick because they become possessed by malicious entities and they need to undergo a ceremony or exorcism to be healed. People who believe in this model experience plenty of evidence of both possessions and exorcisms and from their viewpoint it's true and valid. The consequence of believing in this model of sickness is that you are a victim and need to live in fear of entities that are out to get you. You need to take actions to protect yourself spiritually and can become reliant on the power of the local witchdoctor or shaman

Spiritual Models of Healing

There are many variations of spiritual models of illness but the most extreme are the mirror image of the biomedical model in that they regard the body as illusory and the mind/spirit as the only thing of real consequence. In this view illness is also an illusion founded on an error of thinking (we are created in the image of God and God is perfect, so we must be perfect and therefore sickness is not real) and a return to health is achieved by prayer and the realisation of one's perfect, healthful self. People who believe in this model do experience healing and there are many instances recorded by the Unity Church.

The consequence of believing in this model is that you will not be supported by the dominant culture. If one tries to heal children by this belief and the child dies, the dominant culture will quite likely vilify the parents and prosecute them for neglect as it does not recognise prayer as a valid or effective health practice. Another consequence is that followers of this belief are unable to take advantage of any other healing modalities without encountering censure from their fellow believers.

Energy Models of Healing

Many energy practices regard the restriction of the flow of energy within the body to be the causes of illness and their therapies aim to rebalance the energies through various means. Acupuncture, color therapy, energy balancing and 'touch for health' are all examples of these. One of the advantages of this model is that the therapies don't generally require drugs or highly technical machines so are less expensive than biomedical treatments and thus more accessible. Disadvantages are that the patient is still very reliant on the practitioner for the cure and there is not necessarily much self-realisation as to why one created the energy imbalance in the first place.

Belief Model of Healing

The belief model, as discussed within this book (and taught by the Avatar course and others such as Louise Hay), is that people manifest disease (all their experiences actually) through their knowing or unknowing adoption of beliefs. People get sick because either they deliberately choose to (at some level of their being they believe that this will bring them an experience they want) or they make unconscious choices that attract the illness.

The main advantages of this model is that it underpins and supports all the other models of health and sickness i.e if we choose to believe in demons then we might experience demonic possession and exorcisms, if we choose to believe in the biomedical model then we might experience our body being separate from and unaffected by our thoughts and intentions etc.

Because the belief model supports all the others, believers are free to choose to believe in any model of healing that they feel will be beneficial to them and can deliberately manage their faith in that model and subsequently their experiences.

Another advantage is that as the individual is seen as the root cause of all they experience (through their adoption of beliefs), they can change their experience through changing their beliefs; this gives the power to the patient.

The belief model allows the patient to find their own answer to the question 'why did I get sick?'

Some Questions to consider:

- What model of healing do I believe in?
- Why do I believe in this model?
- Is this model currently serving me?
- Could I consider a different model?
- Am I making up my own mind about my healing or am I responding from unexamined beliefs that I have been taut as being unquestionably true?
- What would it take for me to change my beliefs about health

Chapter 13

Listening to the Body

Life is really very simple. What we give out, we get back.
Louise Hay

The mind-body connection is a two way conduit of communication and effect; not only do your beliefs influence your body but your body influences and communicates with your mind. Communication only happens, though, when there is both a speaker and a listener. The trick in mind-body communication is to listen attentively to the messages the body is sending because it doesn't communicate in words.

The body speaks in the language of feelings and metaphor. At its most basic level the body uses a binary system of feelings in response to our beliefs and actions. If we feed the body with what it needs for good nutrition it will respond by feeling good and content. Likewise if we give it adequate and appropriate exercise the body responds with feelings of well-being.

When we eat foods that are not what the body needs or attach negative self-beliefs to our foods the body responds with feelings of discomfort. Under-exercise and the body will feel torpid and flat. It's a very simple system of biofeedback: feeling good means 'yes' and feeling bad means 'no'.

This binary system of communication is used by kinesiologists (also known as muscle testing or touch for health') who can communicate directly with the body wisdom of their patients by asking questions and then testing the strength of the patients' muscles. They will lift the arm of the patient and a strong muscle response means 'yes' and a weak muscle response means 'no'.

Many of us, however, either don't feel the body's responses or choose to overlook them.

If one ignores the body and continues to act in ways that are deleterious to it, pain is usually the next level of communication the body resorts to. When we overstrain muscles or joints, they hurt. Continual overstraining will lead to chronic pain. Continued overeating leads to painful digestive ailments and continued stress leads to the pain of stomach ulcers.

Eventually, if the body's pain messages are not listened to, it resorts to communication through the medium of metaphor or symbolic meaning by manifesting a disease. A disease can be considered as the body's last-ditch attempt to communicate with us to say something is wrong. Now we can determine the meaning of the communication and take action, or suffer the consequences, which could be disability or even death.

This can seem like a difficult task but fortunately our everyday use of language contains some useful clues;

- Have you ever been really pissed-off with someone and then developed a urinary infection?
- Do you get headaches when things get too difficult to figure out?
- Do some people give you a pain in the neck?
- Are there some people you can't stomach?
- Do you bellyache?
- Do some people have a lot of gall?

We use body metaphors in language to describe feelings because, unconsciously, we understand the connection between the mind and the body.

Louise Hay healed herself from vaginal cancer through listening to the message of her illness and responding with positive affirmations. She is a much respected authority on how the body communicates using metaphor and in her book *You Can Heal Your Life* she lists common ailments and the probable message they are signifying.

As an example, I referred to her book after being diagnosed with a brain tumor. She lists the probable cause as 'Incorrect computerized beliefs. Stubborn. Refusing to change old patterns.' She also offers an affirmation as a means of a cure; 'It is easy for me to reprogram the computer of my mind. All of life is change, and my mind is ever new.'

My initial response to this interpretation was to resist it, after all I am an Avatar master and quite used to changing my beliefs, but when I considered it further I realised there were some ideas, especially around my lack of self-worth and authority, which I was stubbornly hanging on to.

I find Louise's interpretations very useful but take them more as a starting point than gospel. Considering my disease and its manifestation further I began to put together some more pieces of the message my body was telling me. Firstly the tumor manifested in my left parietal lobe and created the symptom of interfering with my ability to read, write and talk i.e to communicate. Further, I noticed that while I was recovering from the surgery I found it very hard to communicate my wishes to the nursing staff. Even when I was in pain from the catheter and knew there was something wrong with its placement, I was unable to   speak assertively enough to have it removed, with the consequence that I experienced pain for some days after finally getting it removed with the help of my wife. Also I found myself unable to ask for pain relief in the night, even though I knew it to be a reasonable request and would expect anybody else to do it. The beliefs I was hanging on to were about communication and my sense of self worth: I didn't think I had the right to say what I needed, and I didn't believe I would get what I needed even if I did ask.

This was further revealed when it came time for me to discuss my treatment strategy with my oncologist. Even though I felt firm in my resolve not to elect for radiotherapy and chemotherapy, when it came time to say how I felt I suddenly found myself close to tears and was reminded of when I was 14 and trying to tell my headmaster why I shouldn't have to play sport. (Sadly, that time I didn't get listened to and was sent back out to the sports field where I was regularly bullied. No doubt this was the source of my self-limiting beliefs).

Now that I feel I understand the metaphor of my disease I am taking measures to change the old patterns i.e using the Avatar tools I have created new beliefs; 'I can easily use my voice' and 'My viewpoint is valuable to myself and others'.

The writing of this book is an action based on these new beliefs. I feel that through listening to my body and then installing new beliefs and taking aligned action, my body won't feel the need to keep manifesting this disease.

What message or messages is your body trying to communicate to you?

When considering your own illness, be prepared to consider metaphoric beliefs that might, at first glance, seem unlikely. If you were not resisting these beliefs in the first place then your body would not have had to manifest a disease to bring them to your attention. Use Louise's book to get a general feel for what your body is trying to tell you and work from there. It's never too late to listen to the body unless you are in the final stages of dying, which is like a divorce between the body and mind after all communication has broken down!

We humans are very good at overriding the messages from our bodies. Consider the habit of smoking cigarettes as a case in point. Smokers will confirm that their body requires nicotine to feel good and that stopping causes their body to feel bad. But it wasn't always so. I bet every smoker can remember their first smoke and the way the body reacted, but they persisted with smoking until the body was subdued and eventually became addicted. Likewise with alcohol. How many times, after a bout of vomiting, have you said the words 'I will never drink again' and then drank again? Animals learn after one negative experience; dogs will never touch a food that once made them sick, in this respect they are smarter than us.

How do you habitually react to pain? Do you consider how you might be causing injury to the body and then change your behaviour or do you reach for the painkillers so that you can continue with the same injurious behaviour? Advertisers will encourage you to take their painkiller as a quick solution to your pain. Treating the symptom is a quick fix but it doesn't address the underlying cause of the pain. Are you in pain because of a lack of painkiller? No, the body is trying to tell you something.

Louise Hay says that the message in pain is guilt, 'guilt always seeks punishment'. If you are experiencing chronic pain then you could well ask yourself what you feel guilty for or why you think you deserve this punishment. There are no painkillers effective against guilt except confession, remorse and redemption.

If your pain is not so chronic but associated with your illness then you might need to be able to live with it. The trick is achieving balance; there's little to be gained from stoically bearing pain but the side effects of high levels of painkillers can become a further burden on the body.

One way to learn to live with pain is to allow yourself to willingly experience it. If you have pain already then the choice is either to medicate it away, resist it (which leads to suffering more) or accept it and experience it willingly. You can do this by letting your attention rest softly on the area of pain and accept the sensations you feel there without your mind resisting or adding any judgements. Have the attitude of an explorer in a new country willing to experience an intense new sensation. It's not good or bad, it just is. Feel all the different aspects of the pain. If the sensation gets too much, take your attention off it for a moment by thinking about something else then go back and willingly feel the pain again. It's like sinking into a very hot bath, until you are comfortable with the heat. Appreciate the intensity of this sensation without making up any stories about it. (ie 'I can't stand this' or 'this will never go away' or 'this headache always lasts for four hours')

Strangely, the more of the pain you are willing to feel, the less suffering you will experience. You might be pleasantly surprised; once your body notices you are paying attention to its messages, it can stop shouting so loudly.

Questions to consider:

- What is my body trying to tell me?
- If I listened to my body, what would I have to do differently?
- Can I trust the wisdom of my body?
- Am I willing to feel my body; to feel the pain and discomfort of my body?
- Am I at war with my body?
- What do I need to do to improve the relationship I have with my body?

Chapter 14

The Attitude of Gratitude

Gratitude opens a crack in consciousness that lets grace in.
Harry Palmer

Every second of every minute of every day, while you are awake, your mind is focused on something so why not make the effort to focus it on something useful? Of all the attitudes one can adopt, that of gratitude is probably the most rewarding. Gratitude makes you feel good, it makes your situation look better and it makes you a better person to be around. If you are feeling depressed or unhappy and can manage to think of even one thing that you are thankful for then you have already shifted you mood in a positive direction.

I aim to start each morning with an attitude of gratitude, and I can find so much to be thankful for even though I have been diagnosed with a cancer with a very bad prognosis. Each morning before I get up I deliberately feel thankful for:

- Having another day.
- The miracle of brain surgery.
- Not being in pain.
- Not having any mental deficits from having brain surgery.
- Being able to get out of bed.

- Being able to walk.
- Being able to talk.
- Being able to feed myself.
- Being able to read and write.
- Having people who love and support me.
- Having work I can do.
- Medical treatment.
- My friends.
- The self awareness this disease has brought me.
- Being alive.

I am sure you will find that if you can genuinely feel gratitude for your life and the conditions of your life, you will experience a positive shift. No matter how badly off you think you are, you know there are others worse than you and for this you can feel gratitude (and compassion for them).

If you have faith in a religious way then you can give thanks to your creator, otherwise just feel thankful. A prayer of thanks is a true prayer; anything else is just supplication or bargaining. The good thing about gratitude is that you are recognising and appreciating all your good fortune, and what you put your attention on becomes more real. So regardless of your situation, every moment you are alive, you have the choice to focus your attention on what is wrong or on what you are thankful for. The first option will wind you down into despair and victimhood, the second will lift you up to joy and grace. It's a no-brainer really.

Once you have created the attitude of gratitude then you can make it more real by taking action: thank those around you for something real that they are doing or just for being them. Deliberately thank or voice your appreciation to others and your gratitude will infect them and they will feel good also. Gratitude expressed is a positive virus.

A question to consider: what am I grateful for?

Chapter 15

Wanting and Choosing

You will not have that for which you ask, nor can you have anything you want. This is because your very request is a statement of lack, and your saying you want a thing only works to produce that precise experience – wanting.
Neale Donald Walsh

Realising you want to live is a first step towards healing but you can want something and still not get it. We are all used to wanting. We are educated in wanting. If you spend any time watching the television you are bombarded daily with things to want and the implied message that wanting is an acceptable state of being.

Wanting doesn't necessarily create the experience of having because it's not a very powerful position. Wanting actually reinforces the experience of not having, because you wouldn't want something if you thought you already had it. If you believed you were already healthy you wouldn't want to be cured. That statement is so self-obvious it can obscure the truth within it: wanting creates and reinforces the experience of not having.

There are many popular books available today, like *The Secret*, which describe how you can create reality by focusing your attention energy on what you want and then it manifests, but creating reality is sometimes not really that simple.

Some people think that what they need to do is decide what they want and 'put it out there to the universe' then they wait for the universe to deliver. I suspect this seldom works. Why would the universe deliver what you are not prepared to do for yourself? You are part of the universe and if you don't take action to create what you want then why would the more distant parts of the universe take action?

Also with prayer, why ask God for something when you have already been given the power to choose? As Jesus said; 'All this and more can you do.'

When you want something you are also resisting not-having this something; wanting is created by resisting not-having. If you want to be cured then you are resisting being sick. The more energy you put into the wanting the more also goes into the resisting and the belief that you are sick, so what do you manifest; more wanting, resisting and not having!

Instead of resisting being sick acknowledge it. It is what it is. Then you can begin to appreciate what health you have, what life you have. Now you are focusing your attention on what is good and well in your life and you can pray to give thanks for the blessings you have and this is what will increase, 'to those that have, more shall be given.'

Wanting is a state of powerlessness unless you move on to choosing. Choosing implies authority and action; you are no longer asking if you can have something and hoping it arrives, you are making a decision and taking action. You are engaging the part of the universe that is you in creating what you chose to experience. This commitment of belief and action sets the whole universe into rearranging itself to conform to your chosen reality.

When you are in the context of shopping you can feel the difference between wanting and choosing. You can go shopping with a want, perhaps a new dress, and still come home with a want because, maybe, you didn't let yourself have what you wanted, or didn't find what you wanted or you thought it was too expensive etc. If you go shopping and choose to have what you want, you come home with the dress!

Choosing to be healthy puts the power back in your hands. You are the decision maker and you can choose how and when you will be healthy. There are many modes of healing and you can choose to put your faith in any one of them, or you can put your faith in a religious belief or in yourself and the healing power of your body.

Choosing also implies action; you do something. To move from wanting to choosing, you must realise you have the power and the desire to act; you buy the dress.

The crucial point is that to be able to choose you must believe that you have the authority and the power to act. If you find yourself wanting, but not choosing, then look for a limiting belief about your authority, power or ability. In the dress example, to be able to move from wanting to choosing you need to believe you have the authority to buy your own choice of clothing and you need to believe you have enough money (money equals power in terms of financial transactions).

To be able to choose to be healthy, or to choose to recover from cancer etc you first need to believe that you have authority over your own mind and body and the power to make a change. We are not generally brought up to believe that we have power or authority over our own bodies or minds so this might be something we need to develop and practice.

How much authority and power do you currently believe you have? You can use the following scale to rate yourself on your ability and power to decide.

Can you decide to (and have the power and authority to):

1. Change your thoughts
2. Change the position of your body
3. Change your diet
4. Change you medication or therapy or doctor
5. Change your attitude
6. Change your automatic responses
7. Change your beliefs about reality
8. Change your current experience of your body or reality
9. Create beliefs that affect your future experience
10. Create beliefs to change the physical nature of your body (or parts of your body)
11. Change mass conscious beliefs about reality
12. Create or discreate your body
13. Change physical reality
14. Change time and/or space
15. Create or discreate time and/or space
16. Create or discreate physical reality

This scale goes from the viewpoint of ultimate creator of the universe (known to many as God) at the bottom, up to the viewpoint of being in a body but not having conscious control over much of your experience. Note; you might put the items on the scale in a different order of creative ability.

The way to progress along the scale and increase your domain of power and authority is to make more decisions. For example, if you find that you easily have the ability to decide at the first four levels (thoughts, body, diet, treatment etc) but have trouble with the fifth (attitude) then you need to practice deciding and changing you attitude until you recognise that you do have the power and authority to determine it easily, then work on the next ability.

Have you ever noticed that to go from thinking to deciding you have to make a mental change of gear? You can spend hours thinking over all the options and wondering which ones are best and which ones have the most serious side effects and how much they cost, but the thinking mind is not actually capable of making decisions. Thinking is great for comparing data and working out solutions to problems but even when all the data has been thoroughly analysed and compared you still need to step out of the mind and make a decision. Deciding is an act of will and will is an aspect of consciousness that can act independently of the thinking mind.

If you notice that you are thinking compulsively about all the possible actions you could take and all the possible outcomes then realise that you haven't decided, and if you think you already have decided then realise that you are not yet committed to your decision. When you truly decide, and commit to your decision, the thinking mind will quieten.

I used to be a very thinking person and my habitual consideration of the merits and potential drawbacks of any particular option used to render me almost incapable of making decisions. Even the question 'would you like a cup of tea?' would give me trouble so I would usually reply with 'if you are making one' which is an abdication of authority. My life ebbed and flowed with circumstance as I allowed others to make decisions for me.

Choosing my responses to my cancer has been a series of difficult steps on my journey to be more responsible for my own decisions. Making decisions on my treatment, on what I choose to believe about the cancer and on how I define myself as a cancer survivor, and then committing to those decisions, has helped me create peace of mind in the midst of this experience.

When you take the step from thinking to deciding you set off a train of events that leads to an experiential reality. As Scottish mountain climber W. H. Murray said;

"Until one is committed, there is hesitancy, the chance to draw back, always ineffectiveness concerning all acts of initiative and creation. There is one elementary truth, the ignorance of which kills countless ideas and splendid plans; that the moment one definitely commits oneself, then providence moves too. All sorts of things occur to help one that would never otherwise have occurred. A whole stream of events issues from the decision raising in one's favour all manner of unforeseen events, meetings and material assistance which no one could have dreamed would have come their way. I have learned a deep respect for one of Goethe's couplets: "Whatever you can do or dream you can, begin it. Boldness has genius, power and magic in it. Begin it now!"

If you consider the implications of the placebo effect as previously discussed; any action you take aligned with your belief that it is curative will create a healing outcome. So don't spend time agonising over which treatment is the best treatment, or which doctor is the best doctor or what you should believe. Make a decision and start doing something that you believe therapeutic and the action will be curative for you. You can keep exploring options or change your mind anytime you want.

Ultimately you are also going to have to choose, i.e decide, that you are healed. Nobody else can decide for you that you are healed, or, even if they do, it won't mean anything until you choose to believe them.

Questions to consider:

- What do I want?
- Why do I think I don't have it?
- What is stopping me from having what I want?
- What can I choose?
- How can I increase my ability to choose?
- What action can I take today that is aligned with my choice?

Chapter 16

Belief and Faith

When you change your beliefs, your experience will change.
Harry Palmer

Faith is belief without any doubt. We can believe many things with varying degree of certainty, when we are totally certain, then we have faith. The things that you just know are true are the things you have faith in. Although our secular society might seem a faithless civilization on the whole, there are a lot of things we take totally on faith; we have faith the sun will come up, we have faith gravity will remain constant, we have faith our possessions belong to us and we might even have faith that we won't spontaneously cure ourselves.

When it comes to the bigger picture, a lot of us have faith in God, a lot of us have faith in science and plenty of us have faith in both. Being given a terminal diagnosis could be incentive to examine where your faith really lies. Do you believe that your death as predicted by science is beyond the power of God to change? Do you believe it's beyond your power to change?

Science is a belief system. I was never taught this at school nor at university where I studied biology for five years. Science was presented as fact; 'this is how the world is!' and I believed it, in fact I loved it. I loved thinking I knew how the universe worked and it has been hard for me to let that certainty of belief go.

After years of indoctrination in science many of us have absolute faith that science is factual, that it is an accurate description of the way the world is. However, we can never know if this is the case, e.g science could also be a definition of one possible reality amongst many which is made real by our collective faith in science.

Sceptics will advise you not to believe in anything unproven, not to place your faith in any cure or treatment that's not backed up by clinical trials. But they are confusing paradigms: faith and science are not in the same realms of reality. Faith is a realm that encompasses science: you can have faith in science but there is no science to faith.

It is not my intention to try and disprove the scientific method or prove your belief wrong. What I want to do is give you some viewpoints that might open your mind a crack to allow other possibilities. If you have absolute faith in science and science is predicting your imminent death then being able to create some doubt in the scientific method or finding a way to decide it doesn't apply to you, could be helpful.

Our mind's like to create a cohesive model of reality so we won't experience too much fear due to uncertainty. We think we know reality but all we ever know is our model of reality. Science is a model of reality and religions offer different models of reality.

When something comes along that contradicts our model we either ignore it or discredit it because it makes us uncomfortable. If what I am saying makes you feel uncomfortable realise this is just your mind trying to assert its model of the universe. Sometimes it's very hard to take on a new belief if it doesn't fit with what we think we already know.

A friend of mine once had an interesting experience. He was riding a motorbike on a long journey and was far from any town when he noticed that his petrol gauge was very close to empty. He said "I looked at the gauge and gave it a blast from my mind that it should be on full." Next time he looked the gauge was on full. In a state of confusion and disbelief he stopped the bike and had a look in the tank; reassuringly it was almost empty, the gauge had broken! My friend was a trained engineer and his model of the universe could not accommodate the spontaneous filling of the petrol tank due to the power of his mind, but it could accommodate the coincidental breaking of his petrol gauge! If the petrol tank had been full, all that he thought he knew about the world would have been thrown into question.

Can your model of the universe accommodate you overcoming a terminal disease and surviving? If not, you need to let go of the idea that you know all there is to know about reality. Give up your faith in the totality of science if it is no longer serving you, or would you rather be right and die?

I have presented evidence of people who have experienced 'miraculous' or spontaneous cures and I have presented ways of looking at science and statistics which can give you room to move, but ultimately it's up to you.

You have faith; it's just a matter of realising that and realising what you have chosen to place your faith in. You placed your faith in either science or your religion of choice or a combination of both. Surely, when it comes down to it, you believe what you believe because you decided to.

You might have experienced some powerful indoctrination as you grew up that dictated how the model of reality you hold should be constructed, but you chose to go along with the indoctrination. Now it's up to you to look at that model and see if it is still serving you. If it is, all well and good. If it is not, then you can decide to believe something different. If you want to believe you can be healed, that's your decision.

There are many forms of belief in God. Many people who profess to have faith in God show by their actions that they have more faith in science when it comes to health issues; they turn to their doctor or hospital for a cure. This is not to say that doctors and hospitals are not manifestations of God, but they are a step away from having faith in the power God has vested in our ability to create health ourselves.

In the Bible Jesus healed through his faith that God had already given him and the people he healed, the power to heal. He says, "All this and more ye can do."

Fourteenth century abbess, Hildegard of Bingen says "God has given me the power to change my ways."

Neal Donald Walsh in his series of books *Conversations with God* tells us that we don't have to ask God and then wait to see if God decided to grant us our wish. He says that we have already been given the power to create and the freedom of choice and that God backs up all our decisions. The point is that God gives us what we believe to be true, which is not the same as giving us what we want.

So if you have faith in a beneficent creator then pray for your health. If you already have absolute faith that God will answer your prayers then pray with supplication, asking for what you want. Otherwise its best to pray in thanks, recognising what you already have and thank God for that. Thank the Lord for what health you have, 'to those who have, more shall be given.'

Some religions eschew all medical intervention and rely solely on faith in God for all healing, Christian Science and Unity Church are two such. They have many examples of people who experienced healing through faith alone. They also have their share of failures (and these are often sensationalised by the media) but so has every form of healing.

How much time do you believe it will take before you are healed?

Our society has a collective belief in process and that things take time but is this necessarily true? If we look we can find evidence of people who experienced instant cures. In the Bible, the crippled man got up and walked. He believed he was healed and he was. Deepak Chopra's description of the patient with multiple personalities whose symptoms of diabetes came and went as he changes personalities shows that healing can be instantaneous and depend solely on belief.

Lolette Kuby describes her own instantaneous healing of breast cancer through revelation in her book, *Faith and the Placebo Effect*. After being diagnosed with cancer she immersed herself in writings of Christian based New Thought and had a healing vision of God which instilled her with the absolute knowing that she was healed.

So why not decide you are healed and keep choosing that reality until you no longer have any evidence you are sick?

If belief is the active ingredient of all modalities of healing then is it possible to dispense with the modality, the pills, treatments and middle-men and go to the source; you and your ability to decide? I realise this is a challenge; perhaps the hardest challenge anyone can face but it seems that some individuals do create healing through their faith alone. What I am describing here is an ideal; a way of healing that is possible if one believes without doubt; as Kuby described it, 'an absolute knowing'.

I admit that when I was diagnosed with brain cancer I didn't have the degree of faith in myself to just decide to be healed so I decided to believe in the effectiveness of allopathic treatment. After a lot of reading and research and experience I now have more faith in my ability to heal myself directly through belief, which I need to do because the allopathic treatment regime of surgery, chemo and radiotherapy are not considered to be a cure.

I believe I don't have cancer any more. I believe I am healed. My belief is not yet absolute faith though. Sometimes I find myself worrying it might come back, after all, the medical literature informs my doctor and me that this disease reoccurs and is inevitably fatal. However, I have no symptoms of cancer and therefore no reason to believe I do have cancer in this present moment. I can choose to believe I am healed in this moment. And in this moment. And in this moment.

Underneath my mind's worrying, I have a confident belief I will survive this experience and will benefit from it. I have decided to view my illness as a learning opportunity created by my higher-self to bring me to experiences I desired i.e self awareness, the courage to say my truth and a deeper experience of love.

If I am right then great, I am healed and won't have to experience brain cancer again. If I am wrong and the cancer returns at a future date I will have the opportunity to experience it further, learn more and again choose to be healed, or I can have the experience of dying.

Lolette Kuby writes that we can all heal ourselves and don't need to rely on any other treatments or therapies. I agree with her that this is possible, but also believe this is a high level of the use of deliberate intention and that many people are not able to function at this level without a lot of support, study and practice, i.e it's a skill.

If we can't muster the mental or spiritual power to decide we are healed and simply discreate our illnesses then we can avail ourselves of collective belief where it is assistive. We experience our own beliefs but we are also connected to the shared beliefs of our tribe and the collective belief structures of the entire human race.

If the collective belief system of biomedical medicine is offering you a positive outcome then you can use it to empower your own belief, if it isn't, then you need to either go it alone or find another shared belief system which will support your belief.

I've never really been a believer in Homeopathy, I hadn't considered it to be hocus but I wasn't a dedicated user. However, because I have discovered and researched some homeopathic practitioners who have a long-term practice and clinical evidence of success with glioma multiforme blastoma treatment I can avail myself of their beliefs and medications to boost my own healing ability. Even though the treatments are sugar pills with no scientifically measurable active ingredients, I can take them with the expectation they will reduce the chance of recurrence of the tumor. I take them for their therapeutic effect and/or as a deliberate placebo.

We are all subject to the beliefs of others, the important thing is to be aware of this and use it effectively. When I received good news from a radiology report showing significant improvement at the tumor resection site, which suggested to me that there was no cancer, I told everybody I could think of; to create the collective expectation within my community that I was going to be well.

Perhaps, as more people learn to heal themselves through faith and belief, they (we) will create a collective belief which will grow in strength and extent so that it becomes easier for people to believe in their own healing ability. Then we will see the healing centres which Kuby predicts where the sick are supported to heal themselves without the use of drugs or invasive surgery and therapies.

If you realise your current beliefs are not conducive to healing then there are ways to change your beliefs:

- You can find evidence to support new beliefs which will be conducive to healing, e.g. read survivor stories.
- Realise you decided to believe your current beliefs and decide to change them.
- Surround yourself with people who believe what you want to believe, e.g. to develop faith in faith healing, visit Unity Church.
- Experience a faith intervention, e.g. go to a faith healer like John of God.
- Learn to manage your beliefs by doing a workshop, e.g. Avatar Course.
- Pray to your God.

Faith is very powerful. Considering Jesus said that even a mustard seed's worth of faith can move a mountain then how much faith do you need to move few grams of tumor?

An interesting question to consider:

If you had to make a choice between these two options, which would you choose; having faith without treatment or having treatment without faith?

Chapter 17

Summary of Attitudes

*Human beings, by changing the inner attitudes of their minds, can change
the   outer aspects of their lives.*
William James

The following table outlines some common attitudes to disease and the probable outcomes those attitudes can create or attract. Note that it's possible to have energy invested in more than one attitude at a time or slip from one to another as circumstances or mood changes. The more energy and attention you have invested in any one attitude, the more likely you will experience the outcome of that attitude. You might recognise you have habitual attitudes that are on automatic, you might also find plenty of evidence to support your attitude, but any attitude can generate evidence to support itself. There is no implication you will experience all the attitudes listed or go through them sequentially. The main determinant of the attitude you adopt is you. You can decide.

ATTITUDE	DESCRIPTION	PROBABLE OUTCOMES	HOW TO MOVE FORWARD
Desire for death	No longer wanting to live or endure the suffering of the physical realm	Depression. Incurable condition. Death.	Meditate on death. Visualise and imagine reasons to live.

Denial	Refusing to recognise what your really believe.	Loss of feeling. Pretence, worsening of condition	Decide to take responsibility for your beliefs and perceptions.
Victim	Blaming and not taking any responsibility. Letting others decide your treatment. Giving up.	Feeling powerless. Ineffective or harmful treatments or procedures. Side-effects.	Decide to take responsibility for your condition. Forgiveness.
Resistance	Trying not to feel what already exists. Compulsive thinking. Anger.	Suffering. Continuation of condition. Worry and fear.	Choose to feel and accept the suffering.
Identification with disease	Using your condition to define yourself, seeking gain through being ill.	Increased certainty in illness. Intolerance and refusal to heal.	Choose to give up the advantages of being ill. Give up judgements.
Acceptance	Willingness to experience existing condition and sensations	Insights. Relaxation and relief. Reduction in pain and symptoms.	Develop your will to decide and act. 'I accept this condition, now I act to change it.'
Desire to live	Aligning ones intentions with reasons to live	Motivation to take action; research cures, take treatments and engage practitioners.	Act on your intentions. Disempower counter-intentions.

Taking responsibility	Acknowledging you have contributed to the creation of your illness	Power to make changes. Awareness of paths to healing. Insights.	Act on your awareness. Visualise.
Deciding	Engaging your will and your power to determine your attitude and your path to healing.	Confidence in own power. Experience and knowledge. Positive healing outcomes.	Recognise and celebrate your gains. Create new beliefs. Increase your certainty.
Believing	Building faith in your own decisions, your power to heal and your own authority. Believing in a medical mode or practitioner	Increase in certainty and faith. Positive healing outcomes. The ability to help others.	Recognise and celebrate other's gains. Believe that others can heal and support them to believe in themselves.
Gratitude	Giving thanks for your blessings. Realising it could be worse and others are suffering more than you.	The recognition of your good fortune. Feelings of well-being. Compassion. Grace.	Empower others.
Faith	Absolute belief in ones' healing power and ability to determine reality.	Health. Life. Grace. Revelation. The ability to empower others.	Abide.

Questions to consider:
- What is my usual attitude?
- What attitude am I in right now?
- What attitude would I choose to be in?
- How can I change my attitude?
- How much control do I have over my own mind?

Chapter 18

Meditation and Visualisation

It is true that the mind is restless and difficult to control. But it can be conquered, Arjuna, through regular practice and detachment. Those who lack self-control will find it difficult to progress in meditation; but those who are self-controlled, striving earnestly through the right means, will attain the goal. What do I
Bhagavad Gita

In all the books I have read and the courses I have researched about overcoming cancer or other diseases, meditation and visualisation are the most often recommended tools for self healing.

If you want to use your mind to help your body heal then having some control over the mind is essential and this is where meditation comes in. Meditation quietens the mind and increases self awareness. Even in normal circumstances the mind can be a chaotic place, and it can become even worse if one is coping with a major or life threatening illness. Quite likely your mind is fervently occupied with making up stories, worrying about negative outcomes, being envious of others who are having an easier time than you, comparing symptoms, commenting on your suffering, complaining and on and on and on. Meditation can help quieten down all this mind chatter so you can focus more of your mind's creative power on your healing.

There are many forms of mediation but they all aim for the same outcome; a quiet mind and expanded awareness. Some meditative practices are complicated and some are simple, some involve saying a mantra, as in the well know Buddhist chant 'om mani padme hum' and some are silent. You can meditate on a sound or on a visual mantra or you can meditate on a question as in Zen Buddhism.

The simplest meditation is to practice mindfulness of what is going on for you internally. Find a quiet place, free from distraction and just rest your awareness on what is happening in your mind. Watch all the thoughts as they arise and as they pass, also notice the gaps between the thoughts and the space in which they exist. If you can keep aware as your thoughts parade past you, without getting drawn into them, you will begin to notice you are not your thoughts but are something greater. If at any time you notice you have got involved in a thought just stop and let it go. You will know if you are succeeding at meditation if you notice you are becoming calmer.

Eckhart Tolle offers a simple meditation in his book, *A New Earth*. His advice is to rest your attention on the energy of your body. Feel for the sensation throughout the body of the energy field which sustains and surrounds it. If any thoughts come up just notice them and then put your attention back on the energy of the body. At first the sensation will be subtle but as you quieten you will notice your whole body is perfuse with life-giving energy.

A very useful meditation when you are experiencing illness is to rest your attention on the parts of the body which are unwell. Give up any judgments and feelings of resistance and quietly feel what is happening in your body. Feel the discomfort and feel any sensations present. Explore how your body feels with this illness. If you notice any thoughts, maybe regrets, fears or hopes for the future, just let them be and put your attention back on your body. Eventually when you feel you have felt all the sensations associated with your illness you can generate a feeling of gratitude or imagine a white healing light bathing the effected body areas.

Visualisation is the deliberate focusing of the mind's creative abilities on images which will aid your body's recovery. Practicing meditation dramatically improves your ability to visualise. Like meditation, there are many ways you can visualise and you will have to experiment to discover which way works best for you. Some people are more visual than others and easily see pictures in their mind in full color and detail, some can't. It doesn't really matter how well you can visualise, it's the intention that matters.

Visualisation can be assisted by deliberate action. I have heard of one therapist who used the space invader video game to help his patients visualise their white blood cells destroying cancer cells. As they played the game on computers they imagined that each time they shot down a space invader they were shooting down one of their cancer cells.

People who are suffering from cancer are often advised to visualise their cancer cells being destroyed by their immune system. I tried this visualisation myself, after reading about it in Bernie Siegel's book, but I soon realised it contains a flaw (possibly a fatal flaw). Considering that my surgical resection of the tumor was reported as a complete removal, I had no evidence there were any cancer cells in my brain. To do the visualisation I had to imagine cancer cells present before I imagined getting rid of them. It felt very counter-intuitive to me to be imagining diseased cells when I had no evidence they were there at all. The only reason to be doing the visualisation in the first place was because I had believed the scientific statistical evidence that cells would remain or re-grow, I had allowed myself to be indoctrinated with a nocebo.

It's probably far more effective to just visualise yourself healthy and free from disease; go directly to the outcome you desire to experience. Any image you can make and direct your attention to, which depicts you as healing or healthy, will assist your body. Visualise your future healthy self doing something very exciting or desirable, for example, being present as your child or grandchild is born or graduates from college. Visualise Jesus telling you that you are healed. Visualise climbing in the Himalayas or visualise yourself giving a talk on your self-healing and creating a workshop to help others.

Dr. Brugh Joy experienced a non-medical healing and gave up his conventional practice to teach healing through visualisation and other metaphysical methods. In his book, *Joy's Way* he has the following creative visualisation instructions:

1. Relax as completely as possible. All tension must be released. If during the relaxation some part of the body begins to tense, pay attention. Identifying areas difficult to relax will help you see where you carry most of your tension in your body, and this understanding may lead to deeper psychological insights.
2. Recapture the memory of an inspirational experience. Live it again. This trains the emotional and feeling areas of consciousness to flood the body with a sense of well-being.
3. As you imagine the happy memory, allow all the good feelings you felt at the time to flood the body now.
4. Know that this feeling and state of consciousness supports the healing process. Direct the flood of good feelings to the problem area. Feel it wash through. Trust that it is going to every cell in the problem area.
5. Visualise the problem (disease) actually improving, becoming less and less, and finally being replaced by pleasure. Don't worry about how this is being done. The body knows how to heal. Your work is to see and feel the problem disappearing, and to see and feel the healing energy flooding in.

6. Visualise yourself being perfectly well. Feel the well-being of perfect happiness.

I recommend a daily practice of meditation and visualisation until, and even after you are healed. I usually wake some time before I need to get up so use that time to meditate before my mind gets too active. First I feel the energy of my entire body. If my mind has thoughts I use my will to place attention back on the body. After some time my mind quietens and I can feel that I am the energy of the whole being rather than just being identified with my mind; I become more of a feeling than an idea. Then I concentrate my awareness on the area of my head where I had the cancer and feel whatever sensation is there before flooding the area with feelings of well-being, gratitude and appreciation. I finish up by creating an image of something I will experience in the future, like holding my grandchild (not yet conceived) and giving thanks for all my blessings. I also use my Avatar tools regularly to recreate certainty in my belief that I am already healed and will live a long and happy life.

Ideally, when we have complete faith in our health and well-being, we won't need to give it so much attention. Healthy people don't spend all day focused on their health.

If you are new to meditation or visualisation and want to experience success then seek a practicing master and study with them. They will easily be able to guide you in your practice of mindfulness.

Questions to Consider:

- Will gaining control of my mind be helpful to me?
- What am I prepared to do to gain control of my mind?
- What do I already do that makes me feel at peace?
- What disturbs my peace of mind?
- What are the barriers that prevent me from creating a peaceful mind right now?
- Is it possible to have cancer and a peaceful mind at the same time?

Chapter 19

Exercise and Diet

It is the sign of a dull mind to dwell upon the cares of the body, to prolong exercise, eating and drinking, and other bodily functions. These things are best done by the way; all your attention must be given to the mind.
Epictetus

We all know that exercise is good for us and now you have a health condition it's probably even more important to get your body physically active on a regular basis.

When I was going through my six weeks of concurrent radio and chemotherapy I began to feel quite disinclined to physical effort of any kind as I was too busy feeling sick and sorry for myself. However, I was reading cyclist Lance Armstrong's book; '*It's not about the bike*' which recounts his struggle with testicular cancer. Lance had secondary tumors in his lungs and brain and his doctors had little hope for him ever riding his bike again or even surviving. When Lance was feeling down and dispirited, he would get out on his bike and push himself, reasoning that if he was able to push his body to the limit then he wasn't dying. Inspired by his example I went and bought myself a bike and made a point of going for a ride every day. Although I felt sick and was very easily exhausted, having the discipline of a daily effort and achievement made a great difference to how I felt about myself, both physically and mentally.

Cycling may not be for you but there will be some exercise that you can incorporate into your day. If you are still fit and able then move the body enough to increase the heart beat and breathing rate: run, walk, play tennis or whatever. If your disease has progressed to a point where strenuous activity is too difficult or painful then take up gentle stretching, yoga or Pilates.

The main aspect of any exercise regime is that it should be good for the body and you enjoy it. There is no gain in punishing your body; it has enough to cope with already. When you exercise, focus on the gains rather than the deficits. Maybe you can't stretch as much as you used to, or you can't bend without pain, or you have lost fitness. If you spend your exercise time focusing on all these losses then it won't be a very healthful session, Focus on what you are thankful for; being able to get outside in the fresh air, being able to walk, being able to breath. No matter how your body is dehabilitated, there are always others who are worse off than you.

Give your body positive attention. You may well feel it has let you down or that your disease process has rendered your body ugly and unattractive, these judgements will not help your body heal. At this time you need to become your body's friend and support person: give it positive appreciation. Have a massage, take a warm bubble bath or a sauna; your body will appreciate the thought.

Considering that we have already discussed the power of beliefs, are there any negative judgments, thoughts or expectations you are projecting on to your body and its ability to heal? Are your actions the actions of someone who treasures their body? Just consider for a moment what a wonderful creation your physical being is: It grew from a single cell to become this incredibly complex form that allows you to interact with the physical universe. It has senses which allow you to perceive, muscles and a skeleton which allow you to move around, a brain to analyse, imagine and create reality, arms to hold another, the power to create other beings and the power to love. You will never own anything as special as the body so treat it with care and respect, it's not too late

Many people experiencing health issues focus a lot of attention on their diets. A terminal diagnosis is incentive enough to get us thinking about changing our ways and changing our diet is an obviously positive action, but how should we change it? If you look in any bookshop or on the internet, the range of possible diets is staggering.

My advice is to choose the diet you intuitively feel is right for you. Either adopt a whole diet regime as described by someone else (in a book, on the internet or in person) or eat what you feel your body requires. You will know what makes your body feel good and what makes if feel heavy, nauseous, flat or out of sorts.

I don't think it really matters what diet you adopt as long as you believe it's doing you good and you get a positive response from your body. One of the main curative properties of a good diet is your care and intention in adopting it. As you select the fresh organic vegetables, as you prepare your special non-gluten dinner or make a fresh carrot juice, you are focusing positive belief and energy on your health.

The point is to make choices and act from a positive frame of mind; if you are begrudging as you buy the special ingredients or bemoan what you can no longer eat, you are playing the victim and your food will be ashes in your mouth. If your attention is going to all the toxins in the supermarket food and the politics of mass production or food miles, give it up, let somebody else deal with that, you need to put your attention on the healthy alternatives you are sourcing from your local organic farm etc. Feed your body what it needs to be healthy and congratulate yourself for doing so, you are taking responsibility.

Of course there is always the possibility of taking diet concerns too far. For some people diet becomes an obsession and can just become another way of negating, mistreating or abusing the body; bulimia, anorexia and fad dieting are sad outcomes of this behaviour. When you are considering your diet be careful you are not planning a regime that will punish the body. Are you being too strict? If you like to drink the occasional glass of wine or have a daily coffee or any other indulgence that isn't allowed (either by your diet or doctor or inner mean identity) what harm will it do to let yourself enjoy the pleasures of life?

Questions to consider:
- Am I taking care of the dietary needs of my body?
- Am I taking care of the exercise needs of my body?
- If not, why not?
- What would I have to change to start taking care of my bodily needs?
- What can I do today to better take care of my body?

Chapter 20

For Caregivers and Loved Ones

*It is one of the most beautiful compensations of life, that no man can
sincerely try to help another without helping himself.*
Ralph Waldo Emerson

If you are supporting someone through the process of a
terminal or serious disease then I take my hat off to you; I
understand what a challenging task you face. Not only are you
supporting another as they meet what is possibly the most
demanding challenge of their life but you have to also consider
how this impacts on your life; how their incapacity makes
your lot harder and how you will manage if they die.

It can be very tempting to put your life on hold while your
loved-one or partner needs so much support but I advise
against this, it's probably really nourishing for you to have
some time and life for yourself, away from your partner and
all his/her worries. A serious illness can dominate the home
atmosphere and I feel it's very important that family life carry
on as normally as possible, after all, that's what we are aiming
for.

Please realise it is normal for you to sometimes feel angry at
your unwell partner or angry at God or life in general. It's

normal to feel let down by the health system or by specific health practitioners. It's normal to feel frightened, unsure and scared for the future. It's normal to find yourself imagining your partner dying even if this is not what you want. It's also normal to wish your partner would get on and die so you can move forward with your life.

Although all these feelings are normal they are not very helpful, for you or for your partner. The best thing you can do is honestly feel and own whatever feelings come up for you and then decide to place your attention on the outcome you want to experience; the outcome that would be best for you and your unwell partner, a hasty and complete recovery.

If that is not what you think is the best outcome then you are probably not the best person to be supporting your partner at this time. It is possible that some people might secretly benefit from having an unwell loved one. If the ill partner used to be domineering and now the caregiver has status or freedom that they didn't previously have or if the caregiver gets ego gratification from being in the care-giving roll then, consciously or unconsciously, the caregiver could actually be a hindrance to a healing outcome.

It would be a real blessing to your partner if you can take the time to honestly ask yourself, 'Do I want him/her to recover with all my heart and soul?' If you are not 100% behind the goal of a full recovery then be honest with yourself and examine your reasons.

If your relationship was less than healthy before the sickness then this occurrence could bring you closer together, but if you are not fully committed, don't stay out of feelings of guilt or obligation as you will not really be helping yourself or the other. Assuming you are fully committed then how can you best support your ailing partner? Apart from all the daily physical assistance he/she may require the most helpful thing you can do for them is to manage your beliefs and attitude.

If you are finding yourself compulsively worrying and fearing for the worst then you need to take yourself in hand and choose to deliberately focus on a positive outcome. Use the chapter on fear in this book to look for your beliefs about your inability to cope, acknowledge them and then create some positive beliefs. Also, spend time using your imagination skills to creatively visualise your partner returning to full health. Together you could make a shared visualisation or shared future goals. The power of two people visualising an aligned goal is much more powerful than the sum of two people visualising different goals.

There is also an exercise for fear and worry in the Avatar will mini course which you can download from the www.avatarepc.com or www.survivecancer.info websites.

If your concern about the future is regarding practical things then take the time with your partner to address these so that they are not soaking up your attention. For instance, if your partner hasn't made out a will or if there are financial matters that need attention then the best thing to do is get them sorted. You might find your partner reluctant to deal with issues that might suggest they are going to die at any moment, especially if they are in a state of denial or resistance about their disease. What might seem to you to be sensible precautions might seem to them like giving up on living but with some patience and understanding they could come around to the viewpoint that it's better for both of you to have these issues sorted. Having a will is sensible for everybody, not just for those facing imminent death so making a will is not the same as deciding that one is about to die.

When I am with others who are suffering I aim to maintain the mental viewpoint that *everything is all right*. This can be a challenge as some things don't seem right at all. When the people we love are suffering, when our children are suffering, it certainly feels like there is something wrong with the world and things have to change, right now! However I find that getting upset and resisting whatever is going on just makes me less able to respond and help so I keep returning to that attitude. *Everything is all right and everything will be all right.* I also hold a strong intention in my mind that a positive outcome is happening or will happen soon.

If you can maintain this attitude as your partner goes through their healing journey then you will be supporting them mentally and spiritually as well as physically. A positive attitude is the best thing you can create to help them integrate their experiences and heal but it has to be real. A pretend positive outlook when you are really scared and negative is not only obviously false to others but it will sap your energy. You need to recognise your fears, either privately or with your partner when they are feeling strong, and then choose to put your attention on whatever real positivity you can muster. Make a habit of finding things to be thankful for and positivity will become second nature to you. Just yesterday I was asked if I find it a drag that I have to rely on people to drive me around (as I lost my drivers license due to having a seizure) I honestly replied that it wasn't a drag as I'm thankful I am able to walk. A friend of mine has just had brain surgery for the second time and is now not able to walk so I really do feel fortunate.

I also think it's important to empower your partner's choices. Sometimes you will think they are making the wrong choice in their treatment but there really aren't any wrong choices, just different viewpoints. The more you can empower your partner's ability to decide the more they will be able to take responsibility for their healing. However, sometimes your partner will act the victim and it's important not to play along, likewise when they are angry or depressed, just maintain your own attitude and love them as the amazing creative healing and loving being you know them to be, soon enough they will find themselves again.

As a care giver for a person facing a terminal prognosis you are facing a heroic challenge, one you have probably not had any training for or (hopefully) prior experience of, so you are going to make mistakes. You are going to feel hopeless and helpless at times and it might seem that what's being asked of you is more than you can possible cope with. Try not to let this get you down; you don't need to know all the answers, you don't need to know what to do or what will happen, all you need to do is be there and love this person as much as you can and know *'everything will be all right.'*

Questions to consider:

- Are my beliefs helpful or impeding to the recovery of the patient?
- On what evidence are my impeding beliefs based?
- Can I change my beliefs to better support the patient?
- What am I afraid of?
- How can I take responsibility for my fears?
- How can I manage my attitude
- What would I gain or loose if the patient dies?
- What would I gain or loose if the patient recovers?

Chapter 21

Alternative Modes of Treatment

A good night's sleep, or a ten-minute brawl, or a pint of chocolate ice cream, or all three together, is good medicine.
Ray Bradbury

There is currently a huge divide between the scientific medical establishment and alternative medical practitioners and this is a great pity and it is probably causing the death of many people. You only have to spend a few minutes researching alternative cancer cures on the internet before you will find attacks on medical science, doctors and drug companies. Writers who support medical science also regularly attack the practices and practitioners of alternative modalities of medical treatment. If this divide could be mended through good will, appreciation and aligned goals then patients could more easily make the transition between the healing modalities.

When I began to research the possible alternate cures and treatments for my condition I quickly became confused by all the different viewpoints and claims expressed. There were so many different and seemingly contradictory options that it was almost impossible to determine what true and effective; in which treatment should I invest my money, time and belief? Which diet is the right diet? Which clinic is getting results that are reliable? Which book has the secret of a miracle cure? Which faith healer has enough faith?

Every modality of healing has its supporters and its detractors. Every therapy has case studies of patients cured and, no doubt, plenty of examples of patients who died. The literature is also sprinkled with allegations of malpractice, stories of doctors being arrested in foreign hotel rooms after administering illegal drugs to patients who subsequently died and accusations of viable cancer cures being suppressed by government authorities.

It seemed to me that the biggest choice I was faced with in the alternate treatment arena was 'what do I believe' and then it all began to make sense to me. People experienced success in the therapy that they chose to believe in. The main factor in their choice and their experience was their belief, not the modality they chose!

Deciding on your modality of healing and the practitioners who will support you to heal are equally important tasks. As we discussed above, the beliefs of your health practitioner can be an important aspect of your healing. If you can gather about yourself a team of caring and experienced therapists then you will be in a better position than if you decide to go it alone.

The value of a good practitioner can not be overstated. From my own experience supporting students on the Avatar course I know that my beliefs and commitment to their success is a very important component of a successful outcome. Many of the Avatar exercises can be done without the help of an Avatar Master but the results might not be so good, especially for someone trying the exercises for the first time. As I have worked with hundreds of students before, I know what a good result is and will encourage a student to push on to get the best possible result they can. Without a guide, students can be tempted to stop before getting a result or can be satisfied with an OK result and not push on for a great result. Likewise, a skilled and experienced health practitioner can bring a depth of knowledge and positive expectation that will contribute to your healing outcome way beyond what you could reach by yourself. Also, if they have witnessed positive outcomes before for your illness then they will naturally be able to pass that positive belief on to you, and sustain it when you go through tough times. It's my advice that the most important attribute to look for in a health practitioner is their manner; do you feel that they are genuinely concerned about you and will they listen to you and respond to your requests. Therapeutic ability and experience is, of course, a very important consideration but if you don't feel fully supported by your therapist then their abilities might not help you.

When considering a practitioner there are some questions you could ask:

- Does this practitioner believe in my ability to overcome this disease?
- Do they have a compassionate and caring manner?
- Is this practitioner genuinely interested in me or are they more focused on selling a product or pushing their cause or cure?
- Will this practitioner's beliefs empower or disempower me (if I take them on)?
- Will this practitioner easily work with practitioners of other healing modalities or does he/she harbour blame and animosity?
- Has this practitioner experienced positive outcomes for other patients with my disease using their treatments or therapies?

Every method of healing works! Granted, every method will have its share of practitioners who are inept or unpleasant and every method will have its successes and its failures but a method of healing wouldn't exist if it didn't help people to heal. Even the methods that are outdated and seem ridiculous to our modern view, worked in their time.

So are some methods better than others? Now we are back in the realm of personal preference, experience and belief. Everyone will have their own belief about which method and which practitioner is best.

I think that a good criterion for deciding the merits of different healing methods is whether they will empower or disempower the patient as the source of healing.

For instance, allopathic medicine is very good at diagnosis and emergency procedures like broken bones and accidents but generally the patient is considered as a passive component of the healing process. On the whole, medical doctors are all too ready to take the responsibility and the credit for their patients' experiences. They see the cures as residing in the drugs or the treatment and not in the patient. You may well experience a cure for a condition through the use of allopathic medicine but it's unlikely you will get any support or empowerment to be self-healing from the process. Many people get treated in a way that is very disempowering within the hospital environment; they end up feeling like broken machines or slabs of meat. My feel is that allopathic medicine is generally for people who don't want to take full responsibility for their health, although everybody's experience is different and one can choose to use allopathic treatments with self-awareness and responsibility.

I find it peculiar that the health practice our society thinks of as the most sensible or responsible choice to make, i.e allopathic medicine, actually engenders the least personal responsibility for illness within the patient. Medical insurance, malpractice suits and prosecutions of people who choose to treat their children through faith healing (and fail) are further symptoms of a society that discourages personal responsibility.

Questions for you to consider

- Which therapy can I believe in fully?
- Will this therapy or practise empower my ability to self-heal?
- What evidence or reassurance do I need to make a decision?
- What do I feel intuitively drawn to?
- What positive (or negative) experiences have I had in the past with alternate health practices?

Chapter 22

Friends and Loved Ones

In poverty and other misfortunes of life, true friends are a sure refuge. The young they keep out of mischief; to the old they are a comfort and aid in their weakness, and those in the prime of life they incite to noble deeds.
Aristotle

Seen much of your friends lately? Well don't take it personally; it seems to happen to most of us. A serious sickness and the thought of impending death are often too much for our friends to handle. Of course our closest friends and loved ones will stick with us (ideally) but for our casual acquaintances, it's unfortunate, but we just make them feel too uncomfortable.

Nobody wants to be reminded they are mortal and that all their plans and accomplishments will be washed away on the next tide. As we, the condemned, walk around, we raise the spectre of death and are therefore shunned. Forgive them because they know not what they do.

Another difficulty often encountered by people experiencing life-threatening illness is that many of their friends and even family members will want to connect with them on a very superficial basis. They will adopt an overly cheerful or positive persona and try to hide their real fear and discomfort. The best thing you can do is respond with compassion and be as real as you can. Everybody hurts and our pain reminds them of their own. In a way we are the trailblazers for those we know; we are gong ahead into the darkness. Managing our state honestly and positively is the best thing we can do to help them.

It behoves us to aim to strike a balance in what we tell others; if we gloss over our experience then our listeners will feel that we are deceiving them and that we don't truly trust or value them. If we take every opportunity to tell our sorry story and download all our fears and concerns onto our listeners then that is an unfair burden for them to carry and they will begin to avoid us. Balance is easiest achieved if you seek to take responsibility for your state, integrate your fears and victimhood and then you will be able to honestly communicate with others without feeling the need to hide or impress.

Those who stick with us through our illnesses, they are angels in human form, not afraid to face discomfort and death and the spectre of their own frailty and loss. In many ways it's harder for them because, when we die, it will be all over for us but their grief will be just beginning.

If you are married or have a life partner who is supporting you in these difficult times, go easy on them as they have a lot to cope with.

Just as we have intentions and beliefs that are less than wholesome; so do they. There will be times when they are impatient and angry with you. Times when they are so fearful for their own loss that they shut off from you and times when their courage fails in the face of the cruelty of sickness. Hardest of all for them, as for us, is the uncertainty.

It's not uncommon for the partners of the terminally ill to experience the desire that their loved one will get on with it and die, then they can experience certainty once more, even if it is just the certainty of loss and grief. It's very hard for a loving caregiver to admit to feelings such as these, to you or to others, so it's important that you can be as honest and understanding as you can be with them.

If your loved ones are having difficulty coping then professional help is a very good idea. If you are bed-bound and require a lot of physical support then hiring a nurse so that your caregiver can have some respite would be a great help. It takes at least two adults to adequately provide long-term care for a bed-bound patient. If your partner is having difficulty with the psychological issues around your illness then encourage them to seek the help of a councillor or other professional therapist.

If at all possible seek to be aligned with your loved ones about the future. I had a lot of difficulty with this when I was first diagnosed. My attention was all on denying the possibility of my death. I wouldn't consider it for a moment and wouldn't take any action that was predicated on the idea I would soon be dead. My wife however had all her attention on what would happen if I died. For her, my imminent death was such a worry it was all she could think of. She wanted to talk about how she could manage without me, what she would need done to the house, where she could live and how she would support herself. Needless to say we weren't aligned and it was very frustrating for both of us.

When Stephanie wanted to talk to me about something that was preying on her mind about my death I refused to listen. Eventually, I realised I would have to allow myself to see things from her perspective and appreciate there were some serious issues which needed to be addressed because I could well be dead soon and she would be alone. I realised I didn't have to feel like I was giving in to mortality to consider what needed to be done. Once I was able to appreciate her viewpoint I noticed I actually live in a dysfunctional way; I live as if I will be a better person in some future time and will finish all the things I can't be bothered to finish right now. The things that needed attention in case I die actually needed attention if I live also. Over the past few months I have been attending to the aspects of our domestic life that are not working properly and arranging them so that Stephanie can manage without me, this has been a real relief for both of us.

Above all value and appreciate your friends and family, but you don't need me to tell you that do you?

Questions to consider:

- How can I help my friends feel comfortable with my condition?
- Am I creating distance from my friends?
- How much attention am I giving to the experience of my nearest and dearest?
- How can I be more loving?

Chapter 23

Why are we suffering from cancer?

A metaphysical view.

There are many theories about why we get cancer; they range from genetic mutations through to environmental carcinogens, improper diet and the use of cell phones and other electromagnetic equipment. I intend to look at the question from a more metaphysical perspective.

First of all, how much do we suffer from cancer? The statistic that is often cited, especially by people promoting alternative cancer cures, is that 1 in 3 people suffer from invasive cancer at some time in their life.

At first sight this seems unbelievably high so I went looking for the source of this information and found it in statistics published by the American Cancer Society[1].

In the period 2002 -2004 the chance of developing invasive cancer over a lifetime (from birth – death) is 44.94% or nearly 1 in 2 for men and 37.52% or just over 1 in 3 for women.

Further information from the same source tells us that 1,500 Americans are predicted to die every day from cancer in 2008 and that cancer is responsible for 1 in every 4 deaths. Globally, 7.6 million people died from cancer in 2007.

The only good news in this deluge of death is that the 5 year survival rate over all cancers in the US is 66% in 2008 which is up from 50% in 1975-1977.

So, from a statistical viewpoint, and assuming that the US statistics can be extrapolated globally, more than 1 in 3 of us will develop invasive cancer in our lifetime and about half of those cases will prove fatal.

What is cancer? As I am not a doctor I won't attempt to answer this question from a medical perspective but more from a symbolic viewpoint.

We perceive our body to be a unique and singular organism but it is actually a colony of billions of cells acting in alignment. Each cell in our body has an individual existence; it is created, lives for a period carrying out its function and then dies and is replaced. This all happens below our level of conscious awareness but is essential for our continued existence and good health. Our very existence is a miracle of cellular co-operation; every second of our life relies on millions of aligned and organised interactions and communications between our cells.

Cells are arranged in groups called organelles and organs and are differentiated to perform different functions, all of which are necessary to the functioning of the organism as a whole. Our cells act with a singular intention; to carry out their individual function for the good of the whole being.

Cancer happens when one of our cells start to act independently; it begins to grow and multiply out of alignment with the needs of the greater body. It's as if cancer cells no longer hear or obey the needs of the body and set off

142

to have their own existence, even though this can lead to the death of the body and therefore their own demise.

Cells don't really have much imagination, when they set off for an independent existence all they know to do is to multiply and so this is what they do, some cancer cells will also continue to perform their specialised function as they spread and multiply e.g cells from the testis, when cancerous, can produce high levels of oestrogen throughout the body.

Cancerous cells have certain characteristics[2]

- They acquire the ability to promote their own growth and they develop the ability to ignore the anti-growth signals of the body.
- They lose the ability of apoptosis (which is a mechanism that allows cells to die if their genetic material becomes corrupted) which therefore leads to unchecked growth.
- They lose the capacity for senescence, leading to limitless replicative potential (immortality)
- They acquire the ability to promote the formation of blood supply (angiogenesis) allowing the tumor to grow beyond the limitations of passive nutrient diffusion.
- They acquire the ability to invade neighbouring tissues.
- They acquire the ability to build metastases at distant sites

The completion of these multiple steps would be a very rare event without:

- Loss of capacity to repair genetic errors, leading to an increased mutation rate (genomic instability), thus accelerating all the other changes.

Using the metaphysical principle of *as above, so below*, we can compare the situation of cells working in co-operation to sustain the body with the similar situation of human individuals being part of the larger whole that is life on earth. There are billions of us living as part of a larger organic system that includes every plant and animal species and the biosphere of the earth. Our species and individual health is totally dependant on the overall health of this greater system, sometimes personified as Gaia.

From this viewpoint we have many characteristics in common with cancer:

- We have the ability to promote our own growth and ignore the antigrowth signals from Gaia (famine, drought, plague etc) and are experiencing huge population growth globally.
- We have the ability to overcome genetic limitations and experience unchecked growth through technological advances.
- We are developing the ability to live longer and increase our replicative potential.
- We have the ability to increase our resource supply above the limits of natural production, (the use of fossil fuels that represent past deposits of stored solar energy)
- We have the ability to invade neighbouring ecosystems as evidenced by the continuing extinction of other species through human activity.
- We have the ability to build colonies all over the world and to exploit every available ecosystem.

My suggestion as to why we are experiencing so much cancer is that we are behaving so much like cancer and that this behaviour is accelerated by our loss of capacity or intention to repair our errors.

The cure for our collective cancer is therefore to realign our purpose with that of the greater being of which we are a part (of which we currently perceive ourselves as being separate from). As a species we act to multiply ourselves at the expense of our environment even though we know that we can't survive without a healthy environment. Unchecked, we will become a tumor that kills the body which supports us. Global warming, natural disasters and resource depletion are the signals from Gaia which are telling us to start acting for the good of the whole rather than for our own selfish gain.

On a society level we need to recognise that other cultures and societies are part of our greater being and that fighting for ideological control or resource use is ridiculous. Does your liver compete with your lungs for blood supply? No, because they recognise they are both part of the same organism. If one country goes to war with another to secure their supply of resources but causes untold death and suffering in the other country, how is the human species better off? Ideas and ideologies which separate peoples are errors of thinking that accelerate our society level cancer behaviours.

On an individual level we need to realise we are members of families, communities and society and that our actions need to be aligned with the good of the society as a whole. Our individual acts of selfishness are metaphorical equivalents of the growth of individual cancer cells.

If we strive to increase our position and acquire exclusive access to resources at the expense of others we are creating ourselves as tumors. We may think this behaviour increases our personal chance of survival but none of us can survive alone, we are all totally dependant on the survival or our communities, our societies and our planet.

We have stopped listening to our intuitive guidance which is always prompting us to act in a way aligned with the greater good and are acting from the viewpoint of personal ego.

We are dying of cancer at an alarming rate, I propose that unless we learn from our errors and start acting in alignment with life itself by striving to ensure that every action we take is for the betterment of the whole then cancer will continue to act to reduce our population. Like our bodies, Gaia has inbuilt systems to maintain health, if we threaten those systems then they will act to curb our growth, (increased death through disease, resource depletion and natural disasters). If we overcome those systems then we will die with the planet.

If, however, we are prepared to change our ways and live more in harmony with the earth, I believe we will experience less sickness and suffering.

A healing visualization

Sit or lie somewhere comfortable where you won't be disturbed for about 20 to 30 minutes. Unplug or turn off the phone, it's a way of prioritising your needs!

It doesn't matter how well you do this visualisation as long as you have the intention to do it fully. Some people can easily visualise in full color and others can't, but the power is in the practice. Complete each step before moving on to the next one.

Relax and feel your body.

Take five deep, slow, breaths and relax a little bit more each time as you breathe out.

Place your awareness on your feet. Feel the bones and the skin and the muscles. Feel any tension or discomfort in your feet and then allow it to drain away and relax.

Place your awareness on your legs from your feet to your knees. Feel the bones and the skin and the muscles. Feel any tension or discomfort in your lower legs and then allow that to drain away and relax.

Place your awareness on your legs from your knees to your hips. Feel the bones and the skin and the muscles. Feel any tension or discomfort in your upper legs and then allow it to drain away and relax.

Place your awareness on your belly. Feel the bones and the skin and the muscles and the organs in your belly. Feel any tension or discomfort in your belly and then allow it to drain away and relax.

Place your awareness on your chest. Feel the bones and the skin and the muscles and the organs in your belly. Feel any tension or discomfort in your chest and then allow it to drain away and relax.

Place your awareness on your back and shoulders. Feel the bones and the skin and the muscles. Feel any tension or discomfort in your back and shoulders and then allow it to drain away and relax.

Place your awareness on your arms and hands. Feel the bones and the skin and the muscles. Feel any tension or discomfort in your arms and hands and then allow it to drain away and relax.

Place your awareness on your head. Feel the bones and the skin and the muscles and your eyes. Feel any tension or discomfort in your head and then allow it to drain away and relax.

If you have an area of discomfort or illness in the body, or a tumor, place your attention there and feel what that feels like. Feel the discomfort of the body in that area. Feel all the tension and disharmony in your body and mind over having this disease. Feel your resistance to having this disease. Let yourself feel all the negative feelings associated with this part of the body and then let them all drain away and relax.

Now regard that part of your body with a feeling of gratitude and compassion. Flood it with as much positive feeling as possible. If you can't do this yet then go back to feeling your resistance until you are ready to accept and be compassionate to this part of your body.

Invite the cells of this part of the body to come into alignment with the overall purpose of your body. Regard them with the compassionate tolerance you would a small child.

Imagine all the cells of your body acting in perfect alignment, every cell listening to the messages of the body and working in accord to produce vibrant health. Imagine each cell getting all the nutrient it needs and all the oxygen it needs. Every cell is being looked after and fulfilling their function.

Imagine your blood bathing every cell and bringing it everything it needs. Feel how all the organs of your body work in harmony to bring you perfect health. Feel what it feels like to be in perfect alignment with your intention to be healed and healthy.

Now put your attention on your family or the people who you spend most time with. Feel any areas of discord or tension within this family. Feel any fear or violence or distrust in your family as people compete for resources and control. Feel how the people are trying to meet their own needs and the tension this causes.

Allow all this tension and dis-ease to dissipate and relax.

Imagine your family all acting in harmony. Imagine how it would feel to have all the members of your family aligned in a common goal of being a healthy family where everyone's needs are met. Everyone gets listened to and everyone is happy and connected. Let yourself feel what this would feel like, feel what you would feel like in this family.

Put your attention on your community or the people who work and live in the same region as you. Feel any areas or discord or tension within your community. Feel any fear or violence or distrust in your community as people strive to meet their own needs and compete for resources and control.

Allow all this tension and dis-ease to dissipate and relax.

Imagine your community coming together in perfect alignment. Imagine all the people in your community acting to create a healthy society where everyone is cared for, everyone gets what they need and everyone intuitively acts for the good of others. Feel what it would feel like to live in a community like this. Feel what you would feel like in this community.

Put your attention on your whole society, culture or country and feel all the tension and dis-ease between it and other societies, cultures and countries. Feel all the suffering in the world caused by war, religious intolerance and selfish greed. Feel the hatred and distrust people have of others just because they are from a different culture or race. Feel how countries are selfishly trying to meet their own needs.

Allow all this tension and dis-ease to dissipate and relax.

Imagine this world with everyone acting in harmony and alignment to create world peace. Imagine everyone getting their needs met, everyone living in peace and dignity, everyone intuitively acting for the good of others. Imagine a world where every child had enough to eat, access to clean water and education and was safe and cared for. Imagine a world where everyone had a function and could contribute to the aligned goal of humankind as a whole. Feel what it would feel like to live in this world. Feel who you would be living in this world.

Put your attention on the whole earth. Feel the disharmony and dis-ease that selfish human activity is creating on the planet. Feel all the suffering caused by our cruelty and carelessness of our animal brothers and sisters. Feel the tension of the earth's life giving systems as we create pollution, foul up the atmosphere and drive animal species to extinction. Feel all the suffering caused by drought, famine and natural disasters.

Allow all this tension and dis-ease to dissipate and relax.

Imagine living in a world where humanity acted in perfect accord with the natural world, where we met our needs in harmony with the needs of animals and plants. Imagine a world where we are intuitively connected with the good of the whole and our every action is based on what will produce the most good. Imagine living in a world where everything is getting healthier and more life sustaining. Imagine our children and grandchildren inheriting a clean, healthy, planet teaming with plants and animals and rich with resources. Feel how this would feel. Feel who you would be living in this world.

Feel how the earth's breath is your breath. Feel how the earth's oceans and rivers are flowing through your veins. Feel how the earth's substance is flowing through your physical body. Feel how the sun's energy flows through and energises your body. Feel how the universal awareness is your awareness.

Take whatever time you need to open your eyes and finish this visualisation.

To help integrate this vision with your life do an action aligned with your body's healing or do something for the benefit of another or take a walk in nature and appreciate your connectedness with everything.

Chapter 24

Death

Of all mindfulness meditations, that on death is supreme.
Gautama Buddha

Everyone dies. Saints die and sinners die. Lay people die and Buddhist monks die. Old people die and children die. The guilty and the innocent die. I will die and you will die.

You know it's going to happen, the only question is 'when?' and we won't really know that until it happens.

In a way we are the lucky ones; we have been given time to prepare, to settle our affairs, consider our life and make peace with our loved-ones. Most people live in denial of their death even though it is the only thing they can be certain of. They live as though their lives will continue endlessly, flowing without interruption from one moment to the next.

We are different; we have been forced to look death in the face. Maybe you just took a quick peak before denial cut in but that glimpse was enough to shake the foundations of your life. If you are anything like me, you would have felt grief and deep loss for all that could have been but is now denied; growing old with your partner, seeing your children grow and thrive, being there for your grandchildren. Grief and loss are not pleasant experiences so there is a strong tendency to shut it all off and strive to be positive.

If we shy away from fully experiencing this unpleasant truth, though, we are selling ourselves short. There is value to be gained from considering our deaths, as the Buddha reminds us: 'Of all the mindfulness meditations, that on death is supreme.'

Fully and willingly considering your impending death is valuable for many reasons. It could help abate the fear of death and make your passing easier when it comes and it can help you get real about your life and appreciate every moment yet to come.

If you are a practiced mediator you will have your own method to go deeply into your death experience. If you are new to meditation then I recommend you find somewhere safe and comfortable and let your mind consider the following statements. Go deeply into the statements until you can own them for yourself, until you know they are true and feel their significance.

I am going to die.

I am going to lose everything I own.

I will no longer have any money, investments, houses or property.

I am going to lose everything I have worked for.

All my plans are coming to an end.

I am going to part from my family and everyone I hold dear.

There is going to be a funeral for me and my body will be there, cold and lifeless in a coffin.

My friends will mourn my passing and then get on with their lives.

My body will stop moving and never do or feel anything again.

I will take my last breath.

My heart will never beat again.

My blood will stop flowing in my veins.

My ears will never hear again, no more loving words or music.

My eyes will never see again. I will never see trees again, or children playing.

My nose will smell no more flowers, fresh bread or the neck of my lover.

My hands will never make anything again, will never caress again.

My feet have done walking.

My body is going to decompose and become dust and ashes.

My mind will never think again.

My pain will be over.

I will have no more treatments or doctors appointments.

I will not have to answer the phone.

I will not have to get up in the morning.

I will lose my abilities.

I will lose my identity; all the things my ego fought so hard to defend will dissolve into nothingness.

There will be no work for me to do.

Nobody will have expectations of me.

I will not be able to help people.

Eventually I will be forgotten.

Who am I when all this is gone?

It is common, at least in literature and the movies, for people on their deathbeds to begin to consider their immortal soul and their relationship with their creator. The priest visits the life-long sinner in his final moments to hear confession and administer last rites, returning the lost sheep to the fold. Maybe, as all our worldly concerns melt away in the furnace of our approaching death, we are left with only the core issues of our being. If you have had a religious upbringing or practice then now would be a good time to consider your relationship to God and review your beliefs about what happens when you die; get a bit of revision done before the final exam!

I have no personal experience of dying (that I can remember) so don't have much to say on the subject but there are others who have a lot to say and their viewpoints can be very reassuring.

Kathleen Dowling Singh has been involved with terminal and dying patients for many years and has written of her experiences in *The Grace in Dying*. It is a very dense and wordy book and explores the transforming power of death. If you have fears, unanswered questions or reservations about your coming demise then this could be a worthwhile read--if you have enough time. Singh recommends that if you are near the end of your life then don't use the time reading her book. She says

'If you are the one who is facing death soon, just put this book down and know you are safe. If you are dying, your mind will come to know this soon. So, go and rest or go and play or go and meditate, so that when you begin to enter the realms of the sacred you will resonate with those realms gently.'

Elizabeth Kubler Ross was a pioneer worker in recognising the stages of the transformative passage from life to death and her books are also worth a read, with the same proviso as above.

Another avenue of research which will yield valuable insights about death are the many reports from people who have had a near-death experience. Many people have experienced being clinically dead and then came back to life. Those who experienced the event consciously have amazingly concordant stories; most travelled along a passage of light and were welcomed by loved-ones or spiritual beings. They report a feeling of deep peace and often feel deep disappointment when they find themselves returning to their bodies. One telling feature of these people is that they report that they no longer have any fear of death, or of life, as they know the universe is a safe place.

It is not my intention in this book to urge anybody to resist death. Resistance is a futile activity and will only cause suffering. Death will come and claim us, possibly sooner than it will come for others who do not have a diagnosis of a terminal disease. My intention is to alert you to the viewpoint that a terminal diagnosis need not be a tragedy in your life, that you don't need to spend what time remains in fear and victimhood. I wish to remind you that you are an amazingly powerful spiritual being creating experiences on the physical plane and that you can use what time remains to the best advantage. Eat, drink, shine up your immortal soul and be merry, because tomorrow we (might) die.

Anyway, enough words about death, it's meant to be an experiential event!

Questions to consider?

- What do I feel about death?
- What do I believe about death?
- Where did these feelings and beliefs come from?
- How can I make my death easier for my loved ones?
- What do I need to do before I die?
- What do I need to do if I'm going to live?
- Are the answers to the above two questions the same?

Chapter 25

My Survivor Story

It is not necessary to change. Survival is not mandatory.
W. Edwards Deming

I was taken to Hamilton hospital mid December 2007 aged 45 due to having a grand mal seizure or fit. CT scan confirmed my fears of a brain tumor, 2.5 cm in the left parietal lobe. I had previously experienced a few discreet episodes of having difficulty talking and reading and the tumor was located in the part of my brain used for language. The tumor was situated near the surface of my brain so surgery was an option and I accepted this course of action without hesitation. Surgery was performed at the Hamilton Neurological unit in early January 2008 and I was out of the ward and recovering at home within 3 days of the operation.

The bad news came about two weeks later when the pathologist came home from his summer holidays, examined my slides and determined that I had glioma multiforme blastoma grade four.

Within the medical literature glioma multiforme blastoma (gmb) is referred to as 'malignant and aggressive' 'grim' and 'inevitably fatal'. The statistical data we accessed gave a 10% chance of surviving 2 years, and that was with the 'gold standard' treatment.

I didn't really want to go and see the surgeon and have confirmed what I already knew but I went and it was not an uplifting experience. After reiterating the statistics that I could expect a 10% chance of surviving two years the surgeon tried to be as uplifting as he could be given the circumstances; he said, 'I know people who have lived with this disease for years.' then he thought a bit and added, 'Well actually, one person and it was two years.' I was full of bravado so I said, 'Well, it's my intention to survive this 100%' and he replied that he didn't want to give me false hope. This was where I realised my hope was my responsibility and that I would have to be the one making choices about my treatment and the possible outcomes of that treatment.

Over the next few months I began to explore the truly amazing phenomena of the alternative cancer treatment bonanza that is available on the internet.

I explored diets and alternate modes of treatment; I read stories of cancer survivors and the tragic stories of the many that didn't make it. I read of miracle cures and I read the newspaper reports of practitioners of miracle cures being arrested when their patients died in hotel rooms in Bangkok (of course these patients had already been abandoned by their conventional doctors after extensive and possible destructive treatments had already failed)

If you have spent any time researching this for yourself, and I bet you have, then you will no doubt have noticed that nearly everybody thinks they alone posses the truth about cancer (or any other dread disease) and that those who profess alternate viewpoints are not just wrong but most likely motivated by greed or evil intent.

Conventional medical doctors discredit alternative practices and they in turn accuse the MD's of being short-sighted, narrow minded, ignorant and in the pockets of pharmaceutical firms.

Further, if you are to believe the rhetoric, these firms and medical organisations actively suppress cures for cancer that are effective and inexpensive precisely because they are effective and inexpensive!

What to believe? This was the question. Should I follow the usual path of conventional oncology and back up my surgery with a course of radiotherapy and then chemotherapy? Actually I wasn't that keen, especially as the scientific and statistical data gave me only a 10% chance of surviving this for very long at all. I was really questioning why I should put myself through it.

I have always considered allopathic medicine to be more about the disease and the drug than the patient and the cure (and their ability to heal themselves) I was also of the opinion that chemotherapy and radiation are a sledge hammer approach.

My resistance to these treatments was added to after reading the 'cancer survivor' stories of others who had managed to clock up a few years of life with gmb. Although they were alive after periods of five, ten and in one case even 30 years after initial diagnosis, their stories indicated continual medical intervention, reoccurrences of tumor growth, resections, debulkings and multiple courses of chemotherapy. Was this quality of life?

Incidentally the woman reporting a 30 year survival rate had a history free from recurrence and gave her faith in God the credit for her fortuitous recovery!

Should I perhaps eschew conventional treatments, described as slash, burn and poison by the more embittered promoters of alternate regimes?

I had already taken the slash option (surgery) and felt better for it. (Perhaps if I hadn't been dealing with a brain tumor I would have been slower to opt for surgery but from where I am standing now I am certainly glad I did, I doubt I would have survived the time it takes to research other options and make a sensible decision.)

It seems that most people go for the standard treatments as offered by their doctors and health authorities and only turn to alternatives after these treatments fail (if they fail). By then, our hypothetical cancer sufferer has been told that there is no hope, their cancer has advanced to a near terminal stage and their body has been weakened by the radiation and chemotherapy treatments – not an ideal state to be in to begin an alternative cure regime.

I reasoned that I would be better off finding an effective alternative while I was still healthy, with my immune system uncompromised by chemotherapy and my brain un-irradiated, but still I was faced with the problem of what to believe.

I could opt for a homeopathic treatment that was reporting an 80% cure rate for gmb (even grade 4) but I had never really put much faith in homeopathy before, though I wasn't against it. I could try ayurvedic treatments as promoted by a practitioner I knew and Dr. Deepak Chopra whose books I respected. I could change my diet, but how; macrobiotic, organic, alkaline, raw food, vegetarian, vegan? Perhaps a combination; halal organic vegetarian?

But how would I get my omega3 fish oil? How would diets combine with the treatments; the homeopathy requires no onions or sour foods?

Should I go for the all grape juice diet? Carrot juice is good. What about apricot kernels? They are banned in the U.S. but used in cancer clinics in Japan and Europe. Had I considered acupuncture?

Friends and family helpfully compounded the issue by bringing me their favourite remedies; my shelves bulged with fennel tea (cleansing), Tibetan gogi juice (good for everything), Himalayan salt (pink and salty) and strange contraptions that supposedly alter the electric and magnetic radiation within the house.

My poor brain was in confusion. What is the truth about cancer, the medical industry and the alternative cures? Is there even a truth? Were there perhaps many truths? Each therapy or cure was supported with either clinical studies or personal stories of diseases cured. What was the common thread through the morass of information, accusations, claims and counter claims?

Then it became clear to me: everybody believed in their cure, or they believed in their practitioner, or they believed in the power of their saviour. The common thread was belief!

It didn't really matter what avenue I chose to peruse for my healing as long as I believed it was the right one. Taking this a little further I wondered; if belief appears to be the main component of a cure then why choose to believe in anything external at all? Could I have enough belief, i.e absolute faith, in myself, my will to live and the healing properties of my body to create a cure without reliance on any diet, therapy or substance?

On reflection I realised that even though I have been studying and practicing Avatar for 8 years (Avatar is a system of living deliberately and creating beliefs from source) I realised I didn't yet have the courage and faith in myself to take this leap.

I have previously managed to self-cure headaches, strained muscles and other minor ailments through the power of my will but brain cancer? There would be no second chance.

So I decided to put my belief into the Homeopathy option (I liked that they actually had a published study in a medical journal, evidence is so seductive). I would back that up with herbal supplements of amygdaline, selenium and omega3 (also the fennel tea was quite nice, the gogi was revolting but worth a try!).

Now there was just the problem of what to say to my wife and my oncologist. Stephanie is a registered nurse and has faith in the medical system. From her viewpoint my decision was stupid and unscientific and just confirmed for her that I was soon to be buried.

Since my diagnosis Steph had also been doing research, consulting with her medical colleagues and reading medical journal articles and they were not inspiring. One of her colleagues had even suggested that the best thing I could do was to get a doctor to write an affidavit that my condition was terminal so I could draw down my life insurance and then spend it having a bit of fun while I could! I didn't like this idea much because the agreement would require me to die in a timely way.

So we had a lot to talk about and it wasn't easy but by the time we were due to see the oncologist I had made my decision clear and Steph was prepared to support me; I would try the alternative approach first and fall back on the orthodox treatments if there was evidence of a recurrence.

The difficulty was explaining this to my oncologist, not that he wasn't understanding or supportive, he was. What I found difficult was maintaining my viewpoint in a formal medical setting to a doctor and in the presence of my wife, a nurse. Suddenly I found it hard to maintain my faith in my chosen course of action. How could I say no to medical science and best practice? I suddenly felt like my fourteen year-old self trying to explain to the school's deputy principal why I shouldn't have to do sports (I ended up having to do sports).

Then the doctor upped the ante by presenting me with new data; a recent study which showed a 50% survival rate at two years for patients with similar conditions to mine (successful removal of tumor, no deficits, relatively young) and I began to get persuaded. Still I stuck to my original decision and my doctor agreed to support me with regular CT scans to check for tumor recurrence even though he thought it was not the best approach (Steph had walked out of the interview by this time)

I left feeling initially that I had made a stand for my health but the further I got from the hospital the worse I felt, I began to feel I had made a big mistake. I sat down with Steph in a nearby park and asked myself, 'Why do I feel bad about this decision?' Then I realised I just wanted to be right. I had a prejudice against the treatments and didn't want to change my mind about them. So I changed my mind and went back to the oncologist and signed up for 30 days of radiotherapy concurrent with daily chemotherapy (Tomodal or Temozolomide) followed by 6 months of further chemotherapy treatments.

The initial 30 day regime was a major disturbance to my life but otherwise uneventful, except that I lost patches of hair due to the radiotherapy and became a bit depressed and tired by the end of it. I responded to the chemotherapy initially with intense nausea but this lessened in intensity and there was a period of exhaustion that kicked in about 6 weeks after the radiotherapy treatment.

At this time of writing I still have 3 months of chemo to go, my hair is growing back and I still have no sign of any deficit or tumor reoccurrence though I will not be having a brain CT scan for some months so as to let the effects of the surgery and radiation to the brain subside.

Meanwhile I am saving the alternative medications as back-up and will commence the homeopathic and herbal remedies once I am finished with the chemo.

In this description I have hardly touched on the mental and spiritual aspect of this time of my life, I will say though that I used all the tools at my disposal to manage my state so I was as honest and real as I could be with what I was feeling and my responses. There were times when I resisted and denied my condition, times when I felt depressed and hopeless and times when I was irritable and unpleasant, but overall, this experience has brought me to a great appreciation of my life and for the people in my life.

I feel the most important aspect of my healing is the changing of the beliefs and attitudes I hold that could exert a negative influence on my will to live and chances of survival. I am confident that if I keep practicing a deep level of self awareness and honesty, keep putting my attention on a positive outcome and devote my energy to the service of others then I will survive, happily, for many years to come. And if I don't, well at least I'll have been spending my time and energy to best advantage and not been feeling miserable and sorry for myself.

Update 24/12/2008

Well it's been a year since my seizure and diagnosis and what a year! I am now finished with allopathic treatment, they can't give me any more radiation and there's no funding available for another course of chemotherapy. I don't think I would take any even if there was. The good news is that I don't have any indication I need any more treatment anyway.

I had an MRI in late October and its findings were inconclusive, which I expected as my oncologist had been telling me for months that they would be. Also, as this was the first post-surgery MRI, there was no previous data to compare it to. The results did show some enhancement in my brain in the area of the previous tumor but there's no telling if this indicates tumor or just scar tissue or healing activity from the radiation etc. I will be having another MRI in January and then there will be the possibility of comparing the two scans to produce more useful data. I'm expecting to see a reduction in the area of enhancement!

Physically I'm feeling pretty good. I still seem to get tired easily but I have gained the muscle mass that I lost during the radio/chemo regime and have been doing quite a bit of physical work. Mentally I sometimes find myself a bit forgetful and have difficulty finding words. Although this is not unusual I do sometimes think it is a deficit from the tumor surgery or treatment, but it's very mild.

When I was undergoing surgery back at the beginning of the year I met three men who were also having surgery for brain tumors and, sadly, they are now all dead from their cancer. As well as the sadness of losing friends, this has also been hard to handle as it reminds me of the seriousness of my condition and doesn't allow me the benefits of being in denial. Brain cancer kills people.

That I am so well, both physically and mentally is a blessing which I am so thankful for. I have no indication I have any cancer or that my life is threatened so I am sustaining the belief I will survive this for many years yet.

I am currently taking a course of homeopathic treatments for gmb though I can't say I am experiencing any definite effects from the medication, possibly an improvement in energy levels, though I did notice them being effective at the occasional times I was experiencing headache and nausea.

(but we know the effectiveness of placebos!) These homeopathic medicines are supported by some very interesting clinical data and report a good success rate with lots of cancers including gmb.

Life for Stephanie, our daughters Rose and Ruby and me has settled down now and we are all getting used to the idea I'm not about to suddenly die. In fact we are all looking forward to an uneventful year.

I recently led a Healing Empowerment Workshop at a local retreat centre. The workshop focused on the power of beliefs in healing and dealing with fear and identities. I had seven attendees and they found the day very useful and had some helpful insights into the beliefs they had about their sickness or healing.

I intend to go to Florida for two weeks this February to participate in the Avatar Wizards course. I feel very strongly this will help me in my resolve to survive and will really clarify some remaining issues. My intention on the course is to gain clarity around my identities which would create a life-threatening illness and align my will to creating certainty in my belief in myself. I notice that sometimes I'm still not doing everything I know I could do to promote my wellbeing so I still have some intentions I need to deal with.

Update 22 January 2009

Good news, I had another MRI and it showed significant improvement on the previous scan in October. Whatever the area of enhancement is, it's getting smaller, so I'm confident it's not tumor. I was going to wait until my result came through before buying my air ticket to Florida but I actually went ahead and bought the ticket two days before the result, on the belief there would be no evidence of cancer.

We are all feeling so relieved about this result, it has lifted the cloud of doubt and fear that has always been hovering around any thoughts of our future. Apart from my continuing health, and being alive when so many gmb sufferers die in the first year, this is the first medical confirmation my treatments are being effective.

Of course, I can't determine if my good health is because of the allopathic treatment, the homeopathic treatment, my belief management and visualisations or because I'm lucky but who cares? I'm not conducting a scientific experiment, I'm striving to survive.

Update 5 March 2009

Wizard was a blast! As well as getting to work with nearly 3,000 Avatars from all over the world I got to make some real progress on my beliefs around my cancer. I worked on my ambivalence to being alive and after a bit of a struggle I integrated my conflicting identities that were creating the ambivalence to my life. What an amazing feeling! This left me in a state of amazement and awe and realising that I chose to be alive and that I choose to keep being alive. I felt so connected to everything and inspired to keep on living and loving.

Update 20 October 2009

Not so good news. In July I started to get seizures and MRI confirmed that the tumour had grown back so I returned to hospital for another craniotomy. The surgery went very well; I was admitted to hospital on a Thursday, went into theatre on

Friday morning and was discharged on Sunday afternoon. I was feeling pretty pleased with myself (and with the surgery team, I do appreciate that they were very involved) however I overdid things and got a swell head, literally. About two weeks after the surgery I had another seizure and began to get a lot of confusion and drowsiness. I returned to the neurology ward and went back on steroids to try and get the swelling down. I am over the steroids now but I have had a couple of seizures since the surgery and it appears that they might be ongoing unless my brain settles down or the medication begins to have an effect.

Steph and I were both disappointed with the recurrence and experienced a whole new bout of fear and loathing. I am still struggling with my brain in terms of comprehension and talking. I find I can read but only very slowly and I don't take in much information. My memory is appalling and my conversation skills appear to be compromised, well I think they are, so often I can't find the word I am wanting to say. However, My language skills cant be that compromised as I was involved in a play just recently; Twelve Angry Men. This was my first time ever in armature theatricals and I was already learning my role as Juror 11 when I discovered that I had the tumour recurrence, I took a week out from learning my script to have the brain surgery and then got right back into it. The show was a great success and I remembered my lines most all the time.

Update 29 November

The tumour has been growing in my head. I have been offered a third round of surgery but have declines: I can't see that a continual process of brain removal being a viable future. I'm taking steroids daily to reduce the effects of the swelling and maintain a sense of normality in my life. I have felt very scared and negative, believing that my death is inevitable (which it is) and immanent. However, after spending a few days at the November Avatar course in Auckland, where I spent the time exploring my intention to be at peace with my life, I felt much more centred and managed to be appreciative of my lot.

It is altogether likely that this recurrence of the tumour will cause my death and within a period of months much rather than years. It is not the future that I choose to experience, but I will experience whatever comes with the most grace and gratitude I can muster. I'm not taking any specific treatments for my condition except regular meditations and a deliberate viewpoint that whatever is happening is all OK. My aim is to make peace with the tumour and the creation of the tumour and the unknown workings of the divine in my life. I am sorry if I am not making myself very clear with this writing but it is difficult for me to put my words together in a way that reflects my thoughts.

Currently I am aiming to be health for Christmas and I have a few goals for the next year: to be well for a local 4 day men's retreat in March and the Avatar integrity course in Australia in April. Good luck to me!

Copyright Acknowledgments

Resources

www.survivecancer.info

Use this online resource to gain more information on how to create your reality as a survivor.

- Join the survivor forum
- Share your survivor story
- Connect with other survivors
- Inspirational book resources
- Useful survivor and cancer links

Healing Empowerment Workshops

Join David for informative and empowering workshops and be guided through all the exercises covered in this book. For information visit www.survivecancer.info or email david@survivecancer.info

For information on the Avatar course and course schedule visit www.avatarpacific.com www.avatarepc.com or Email David

New Zealand Cancer Society

National office; http://www.cancernz.org.nz/

For information on cancer support groups, advocacy and cancer information.

www.planetcancer.org

Young adults with cancer forum and information

www.ingramcontent.com/pod-product-compliance
Lightning Source LLC
Chambersburg PA
CBHW072141270326
41931CB00010B/1837